MARATHON

REVISED AND UPDATED FIFTH EDITION

THE ULTIMATE TRAINING GUIDE

MARATHON

REVISED AND UPDATED 5TH EDITION

THE ULTIMATE TRAINING GUIDE:
ADVICE, PLANS, AND PROGRAMS FOR
HALF AND FULL MARATHONS

HAL HIGDON

Contributing Editor,
Runner's World

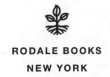

RODALE BOOKS

NEW YORK

The material in this book is for informational purposes only and not intended as a substitute for the advice and care of your physician. As with all new exercise or dietary programs, the fitness program described in this book should be followed only after first consulting with your physician to make sure it is appropriate for your individual circumstances. Do not take risks beyond your level of experience, aptitude, training, and fitness. The author and the publisher expressly disclaim responsibility for any adverse effects that may result from the use or application of the information contained in this book.

The carbohydrate-rich foods list on pages 220–222 was adapted from *Nancy Clark's Sports Nutrition Guidebook* by Nancy Clark with permission from the author.

Library of Congress Cataloging-in-Publication Data
is available upon request.

ISBN 978-0-593-13773-4
Ebook ISBN 978-0-593-13774-1

Printed in the United States of America

Book design by Meighan Cavanaugh
Cover design by Sarah Horgan
Cover photograph by Zamora A/Getty Images

10 9 8 7 6 5 4

Fifth Edition

For our three children and
our nine grandchildren

CONTENTS

TRAINING PROGRAMS

WARM-UP

WELCOME TO MY MARATHON WORLD

New runners, old runners, fast runners, slow runners. They flowed past my booth, many of them stopping to say hello, to thank me for a training program just completed, others drifting by, eyes wide open, as though caught in a riptide that would carry them to their appointment with the marathon the next day.

I was seated in a booth at the expo a day before the Bank of America Chicago Marathon, signing autographs, posing for photos, answering questions. When someone asks for a last-minute tip, I usually say, "Start slow."

And often add, "Finish fast."

If there is a theme to this book, the fifth edition of *Marathon: The Ultimate Training Guide*, it is those two words: *Finish fast.* But split that phrase in two. The first goal of any runner should be: *Finish!* Get to the finish line (after 26 miles 385 yards of running). Cross that line. Accept the medal handed to you or hung around your neck by a volunteer. And accept gracefully all the congratulations you will receive over the next hours and days and weeks and maybe even years. But *Finish!* That should be the immediate goal of anybody reading this book, but particularly first-time runners: *Finish!*

But next, *Finish fast!* Run to the best of your ability. Nothing wrong, after a slow first marathon, with training a little harder, setting your goals a little higher, planning on running a little faster, setting a PR, which veteran runners will tell you stands for *personal record*, the fastest you have run for any specific distance. And for those looking for the ultimate challenge: Attain a BQ. Again, that's runner jargon for *Boston qualifier*, since you can qualify for and run the prestigious Boston Marathon only if you better the strict time goals of the Boston Athletic Association (BAA).

Among the 111 marathons I have run, 18 were at Boston. My biggest achievement was 1964 when I placed fifth overall, first American. In case you're wondering why you should buy this book, why you should believe what I write, why you should follow one of the many training plans herein, trust me. I have learned something from each of those 111 marathons, and I want to share that knowledge, helping you to finish your first marathon and helping you to run faster in your next marathon and marathons to come.

So welcome to my marathon world. And it is a busy and crowded world, populated by millions of runners worldwide. (One study by RunnerClick covered 784 marathons in 39 countries between 2014 and 2017 and identified 2,907,293 runners.) Among the world's largest marathons, consider the Chicago Marathon. I identify with Chicago because my wife and I were born in that city. Among my 111 marathons, I won four overall. One of those victories was the Windy City Marathon, a precursor race for the current Chicago Marathon. That's not as great an accomplishment as you might think; probably only a couple dozen runners participated in that race, which followed a back-and-forth course along the lakefront. Running had not yet become a mass participation sport. Shift to 2018, when 44,610 runners finished the Chicago Marathon. That's *finishers*: not entrants, not starters, but *finishers!* Race organizers also estimated that 1.7 million spectators lined the course, cheering those runners from sidewalk vantage points. I was one of those cheering, not running that day, watching our grandson Wesley run the race. I shift easily from competitor to spectator and back to competitor, and I suspect most runners do the same.

MARATHONS ARE BIG AND BIGGER

Chicago is big, but so are many other marathons around the world. The New York City Marathon (the world's largest marathon) boasted 52,812 finishers in 2018; the London Marathon had 40,255. The total number of marathon finishers in American marathons, according to Running USA, topped half a million in 2010 and has been consistently above that number since that year, the record being 550,600 in 2014.

But in 1993, a quarter century earlier, the field at Chicago numbered only 5,491. Running was big, but it was getting bigger. I consider the year 1993 significant. In that year, Rodale Press, the publishers of *Runner's World*, published the first edition of the book you now hold in your hands, *Marathon: The Ultimate Training Guide*. The book featured a red cover with a photograph of a dozen or so elite men (no women) charging off the starting line.

A half-dozen years later, in 1999, the book had sold enough copies and the sport had changed sufficiently to justify an updated second edition. Its white cover featured a number of midpack runners crossing the finish line in the New York City Marathon, one of whom was a well-known Italian pop-music singer, Johnny Paoli. (Believe it or not, Rodale's photo editors did not know the runner's identity when they selected the shot.)

By 2005, *Marathon: The Ultimate Training Guide* had established itself as one of the bestselling books for runners training for marathons. More changes in the sport justified a third edition. Its red-and-white cover showed a pastiche of runners, slow and fast, including Svetlana Zakharova of Russia winning the prestigious Boston Marathon. Yes, the sport had come a long way from the fast men on the cover of the first edition to the fast woman on the cover of the third. (The RunnerClick survey

mentioned earlier identified the United States as having the highest percentage of women finishers, with 45.7 percent.)

This trend would continue. The black-covered fourth edition, published in 2011, offered a mix of men and women. Standing at the front
of the starting line with the men were Paula Radcliffe of the UK, holder
of the world record, and Deena Drossin Kastor, holder of the American
record for the marathon.

Each of the first four editions as well as this, the fifth edition, featured
a major update on my part, not merely a reprint, but a rewrite. The focus
of each of those editions shifted somewhat as the sport shifted. I gathered
much of the information for the first edition from questionnaires sent to
marathon coaches and follow-up interviews with those same individuals.
Indeed, the cover featured the subtitle *Strategies from 50 Top Coaches.*

By the time of the second edition, I had become more involved in
coaching midpack runners, serving as both training consultant for the
Chicago Marathon and coach for a class of local runners preparing for
that race. The class attracted as many as three thousand runners who met
on weekends at various locations in and around the city. One weekend I
would meet with runners in town, doing long runs along the lakefront;
the next weekend I might appear at one of the class's suburban locations
in Palos Park, Glen Ellyn, or Lake Zurich.

As we moved into the new millennium, I shifted my attention to providing training programs and answering questions for runners online,
both on my popular website, halhigdon.com, and on what came to be
known as my Virtual Training Bulletin Boards. The third edition featured quotes and stories from and about members of my online "V-Team."

When it came time for Rodale to offer a fourth edition, the explosion
of the Internet allowed me to expand my reach to well beyond the suburbs
of Chicago. Whereas I used to meet in person with members of the Chicago training group, time restraints forced me indoors, where my portal
to the training programs of runners became Facebook: a "friend" page
limited to five thousand individuals, but also a "fan" page that attracted
that many and more individuals, many of whom would surf through my

corner of the Internet daily to check out the "Tip of the Day" I posted each morning. Many of the quotes about running used in the fourth edition came from runners I knew mostly through my computer.

WELCOME TO THE FIFTH EDITION

Now for the fifth edition, I find that many, if not most, of my followers now meet me on Twitter. They want their information now, and they want it short and snappy. And rather than from the Chicago suburbs, they come from Munich, Melbourne, or Mumbai. Many of the quotes used in this fifth edition come from runners I know only by a first name or an anonymous handle.

All of these groups—coaches, in-person runners, and online runners—provided the research base for this fifth edition. According to figures from Running USA in 2016, halhigdon.com was the eleventh most visited running website in the world, with two million visitors a year; I also was the third most visible running personality, according to a *Runner's World* survey. Google the words *marathon training* (as I just did) and you will encounter 426,000 results, with my training programs at the top of the list.

Admittedly, not every search for marathon training help will lead you to useful advice—thus the purpose of this fifth edition: to serve as a gateway for those seeking to conquer the 26 miles 385 yards of the marathon; also, to recognize that the sport has continued to change in the nearly decade since the fourth edition.

One major change is the expansion of ultramarathons (races longer than 26.2 miles), many of them off-trail over incredibly difficult courses. You'll find a new chapter on ultramarathons that includes training programs for those doing 50K and 50-mile races. Another all-new section is the "BQ" (Boston qualifier) section, encapsulating the difficulty in running a qualifying marathon fast enough to enter that iconic race. I've included a list of ten marathons that provide the most qualifiers. No surprise that Boston itself sits on the top of that list.

Thus, I offer you this fifth edition of *Marathon: The Ultimate Training Guide*, reflecting the sport as it exists today. I want to show you the way to a comfortable finish if you are running your first marathon or to an improved performance if you've already gone the distance, but are back again. Please join me on the starting line.

—*Hal Higdon,*
Long Beach, Indiana

1

The Mystique of the Marathon

Running 26 Miles 385 Yards Is a Humbling Experience

What would we do for fun if the Persians in 490 BC had won the Battle of Marathon? This thought occurred to me while I was in Greece several years ago to celebrate the 2,500th anniversary of that battle—and the legendary run from Marathon to Athens by Pheidippides, who announced, "Rejoice, we conquer!" and immediately died.

That legend—and it is more legend than historical fact—inspired a race in 1896 at the first modern Olympic Games over approximately the same route from the plains of Marathon on the Aegean Sea to the Olympic stadium in downtown Athens. Only seventeen runners participated in that first race; twenty thousand runners appeared more than a century later for the anniversary celebration. By then, similarly long races with that many runners and more had become common throughout the world. Races that, by the way, are called *marathons*, that term having conveniently taken hold as a description of a running race precisely 26 miles 385 yards long. (More on that later.)

Not everybody understands the drive that causes hundreds of thousands of runners each year to punish themselves and train for months for the seemingly dubious pleasure of running 26 miles 385 yards. One year at the Twin Cities Marathon, approximately 8 miles into the race, I over-heard a woman in the crowd comment: "To think they paid to do this."

I understood what she meant. Twenty-six miles is a long way. Add-ing 385 more yards seems to make the distance even longer and fur-ther confuses people who do not understand what motivates us to run marathons. "How far was that marathon?" they ask after we show up at the office on Mondays with medals hanging around our necks, limping but with smiles on our faces. Despite the rising popularity of big-city marathons, not everybody knows—or understands—why the distance is a precise (but foolish) 26 miles 385 yards. Even thinking about run-ning that far takes a certain amount of endurance. And courage. And maybe even arrogance. Yet somehow those of us who call ourselves marathoners do it again and again and again.

> **It is not merely the race itself but also the preparation that goes into the race.**

The woman's comment at Twin Cities failed to disturb me at the time. First of all, I thought there was some truth to what she said. Second, I was too busy running as fast as I could to worry about what the spectators were thinking.

Only later would her remark begin to haunt me. It was obvious that she failed to compre-hend the mystique of the marathon and why running such a quirky dis-tance appeals to so many otherwise normal people. How do you fully explain to friends and family the joy and pain that go into running 26 miles 385 yards?

I still remember another woman who showed up at my booth at the Chi-cago Marathon expo one year and immediately started crying. She could not talk. She made a few hand gestures in an attempt to cover her embar-rassment but still failed to stem the flow of tears. I smiled—tolerantly. I told her to relax. I knew the reason for her emotional breakdown.

She was about to run her first marathon.

Tears are common when it comes to the marathon. And they are not tears of pain; they are tears of joy. Some runners shed tears crossing the finish line. I did so once myself after finishing fifth (first American) at the Boston Marathon with a time so fast I knew I never again would come close to duplicating it, because never again would I be able to summon the will to train as hard as I had for that one peak performance.

RECOGNIZING THE REAL YOU

"The marathon can humble you," Bill Rodgers, who won the Boston and New York City marathons four times each, once said. Boston Billy meant that sometimes even the best runners crash for reasons not easily explainable to family or friends—or themselves. It happened to him in the middle of that span of victories, when he failed to finish one year at Boston after running in the lead much of the way. But the marathon can humble you in many ways. The classic long-distance race can expose all your nerve endings and bring you closer to recognizing the real you, all flaws and virtues on the surface. Whether or not the woman who cried standing before my booth realized that fact, she was displaying a humbling emotion not uncommon among marathoners.

The tears subsided. She made an unnecessary apology and thanked me for the training program that after 18 weeks had altered her life. She bought a copy of one of my books as a gesture of thanks, came around the desk, gave me a hug, and posed for a cellphone picture. She thanked me again and, eyes still moist, disappeared into the crowd of runners flowing past my booth.

I never saw her again. I never got the crying woman's name. I never found out how she did in the race, her time, whether it matched her expectations. I never learned what motivated her to run what most certainly was a First Marathon (caps intended). I never learned whether she cried again crossing the finish line, although I suspect she did. And at the starting line, too. And maybe a couple of times en route. And maybe while describing the experience to friends and relatives after. I never learned whether she ran a second marathon, or a third, or a fourth, or more.

Many runners have achieved success using my training programs after reading this book or discovering those programs online. I estimate that I've coached more than a half million marathoners, based on sales of this book and visits to my website, halhigdon.com. One woman who stopped by my booth at the Indianapolis Monumental Marathon said she had used my Novice 1 program in thirteen consecutive marathons. But that is not the record for loyalty. Some months after that, while I had dinner in the Plaka after the Athens Marathon in Greece, a woman at a nearby table shouted a greeting. She claimed to have used me as coach for all of her marathons—and she had just finished number fifty-one!

The marathon has been an important part of my life. As a younger runner, I focused my training on making the Olympic team and winning the Boston Marathon—understandable goals. Even though I failed to achieve them, I came close enough to make the quest worthwhile.

As I aged, I often chose more quixotic goals to keep myself moving from day to day and year to year. Sometimes these goals were outside the competitive arena. One summer, my best friend, Steve Kearney, and I decided to run the length of the state of Indiana, some 350 miles. Steve formerly taught and coached at Chesterton High School in Indiana. Like me, Steve is certifiably insane. We convinced eight other runners to join us on what became a 10-day trek from the Ohio River to Lake Michigan. When people asked afterward why we wanted to do such a crazy stunt, Steve and I would shrug and say, "It seemed like a neat thing to do."

SELECTING GOALS

Not everybody who arrives at the starting line of a marathon will have motivated himself or herself by choosing such far-reaching goals as running the length of a state, not even a small state like Rhode Island. Indeed, a large percentage of people entering the most popular marathons are running their first marathon—and it may turn into their only marathon. Thirty-six percent of those who run Chicago each year are first-timers. Nevertheless, each one of those nouveau marathoners will have chosen goals as carefully as I have chosen mine.

For most of them, the goal is simply to finish the 26 miles 385 yards. And that is how it should be. But those of us who have been running for more than a few years often choose different goals. We want to run marathons in all fifty states. We want to run marathons on all seven continents. If you follow my advice and run your first marathon in a sensibly slow time aimed mainly at getting yourself to the finish line, you may want to pick bettering that time as a goal for your second or third marathon.

Certain numbers contain their own magic; thus, runners attempt to break 6 hours or 5 hours or 4 hours. To be asked your time for the marathon and be able to begin your answer by saying "three" puts you in an almost elite, ego-building category, even if your time was 3:59:59. Respond with a time that begins with "two," and if the person asking the question is also a marathoner, his eyebrows will rise and his jaw will drop. I know because I possess a marathon personal record of 2:21:55, and I see the reaction of people when I tell them my time: *"What planet were you born on?"*

You can run 5K races until your dresser drawers overflow with T-shirts, but it is not quite the same as going to the starting line of a marathon.

That may sound fast—and it was in its day—but, consider this: If I were able to re-create that time today (as I write this chapter), I would finish nearly 3 miles behind today's elite runners. That's the men; I would also finish more than a mile behind the fastest women. Among the men, Kenyan Eliud Kipchoge ran 2:01:39 at the 2018 Berlin Marathon. Among the women, Brigid Kosgei of Kenya ran 2:14:04 at the 2019 Chicago Marathon.

Finishing times mean much less to me today than they did decades ago, and it is not entirely because I know my best times are behind me. Most important is just being there, doing that. For me and for so many other experienced runners, it is not merely the race itself but also the preparation that goes into the race: the steady buildup of miles, the long runs on Sundays, the inevitable taper, the ceremonial aspects of the total experience. Two positive aspects of marathoning are that (1) it provides focus for your training and (2) it offers a recognizable goal. The increasingly popular half marathon also does that, but not quite as much.

If you love to run, you appreciate the motivation the marathon provides for those long Sunday runs and those fast midweek track workouts. Marathon training focuses the mind, and that may be the best excuse for racing this distance.

I continue to work out daily, not to improve my times at the marathon and at other distances, but simply because I enjoy being physically active. When possible, I pick scenic courses that provide me with enjoyable sights and sounds. Races become just a by-product of the marathon lifestyle.

THE MARATHON LIFESTYLE

Another positive by-product of marathons is improved health. Marathon running has the potential to significantly increase your life-span and positively impact the quality of your life. Again, it is not so much the running of the race that affects your health but the lifestyle changes that often accompany the commitment to run a marathon. To become a successful runner/marathoner, you need to (1) follow a proper diet, (2) eliminate extra body fat, (3) refrain from smoking and heavy drinking, (4) get adequate sleep, and (5) exercise regularly. Epidemiologists such as the late Ralph S. Paffenbarger, MD, who analyzed the data of Harvard University alumni, have determined that these five lifestyle changes possess the potential to add years to our lives. In fact, Kenneth H. Cooper, MD, the renowned author of *Aerobics*, suggested that researchers at his Cooper Institute in Dallas believe that the proper combination of diet and exercise plus preventive health maintenance can extend life by as much as six to nine years!

When Ken told me this while I was interviewing him for an article in *Runner's World*, at first I didn't believe him. But he had the numbers, the tens of thousands of individuals (runners and nonrunners) who have served as his patients and also his research base. I'm part of Ken's database, and I can say with pride, but also some sorrow, that I've outlived my father by twenty years; my mother, by five years. And still counting.

But the marathon lifestyle is not without some risks. Running is a stressful activity. Running for 26-plus miles makes it even more stressful. In warm-weather conditions, the stress can be extreme if runners do not slow down and drink sufficient fluids during the race. "We're unquestionably more at risk the hour a day that we run," says Paul D. Thompson, MD, director of preventive cardiology at Hartford Hospital in Connecticut and a 2:28:15 marathoner, "but the other 23 hours in the day, we are much less at risk. In balance, you're much safer exercising than not exercising." In fact, one study by Dr. Donald A. Redelmeier, professor of medicine at the University of Toronto, as reported in the *British Medical Journal*, suggests that we are much safer running 26.2 miles on a road than we would be driving that same road in a car!

RISKY RUNNERS

How risky is running? Paul D. Thompson, MD, concedes that runners incur some risk. While delivering a lecture titled "Historical Concepts of the Athlete's Heart" at the annual meeting of the American College of Sports Medicine (ACSM), Dr. Thompson cited several seminal studies quantifying the risks of exercise, beginning with one of his own that suggested sudden cardiac death is seven times more likely during jogging than at rest. He

(continued)

estimated the incidence as one death annually for every 15,240 healthy joggers.

Another study, published in the *New England Journal of Medicine*, offered similar statistics: one cardiac arrest for every eighteen thousand previously healthy men. A national fitness chain, however, claimed one death per eighty-two thousand members or per 2.6 million workouts.

"There is cardiac risk from exercise," concedes Dr. Thompson, "but this risk is small and, at least in adults, most common among those who exercise least."

What safety precautions should you take before becoming a runner or signing up for your first marathon? If you are older than thirty-five, if you are overweight, if you smoke or once smoked, if you have high blood pressure or high cholesterol, if you follow a fast-food diet, if you have a family history of heart attacks, or if you don't already exercise, then your degree of risk is greater than that of someone without those *if*s. Check with your family physician before starting to run. And once out the door, follow a sensible training program, such as those in this book.

There is a mystique about running a marathon, no doubt about it. You can run 5K races until your dresser drawers overflow with T-shirts, but it is not quite the same as going to the starting line of a marathon. And although the half marathon serves as a useful interim goal for runners new to the sport, finishing 13.1 miles is not quite the same as finishing 26.2. Marathons, on average, seem to be bigger and more important events than 5K or half marathon races, even when those shorter-distance events attract large fields. (The Peachtree Road Race in Atlanta, a 10K, featured nearly 60,000 finishers in 2018.)

Arrive several days in advance of a marathon and you know you are at a Big Event, regardless of how many people are entered. Maybe the excitement is partly anticipation among those who have entered. Each runner has committed so many miles in training for this one event that the race takes on a level of importance above and beyond the ordinary, regardless of the size of the field. One year I visited Toledo, Ohio, to lecture the night before the Glass City Marathon, with its field of about one thousand runners. Compared with marathons in New York or Chicago or London or Berlin, with their fields near forty thousand runners, that is pretty small potatoes. Yet despite Glass City's relatively small field, I could feel the same premarathon excitement around me as I spoke. People often talk about the "glow" surrounding pregnant women. There is a similar glow around expectant marathoners. Many of them have devoted, if not 9 months, at least 18 weeks of preparation for their big day. All the people in my audience at Toledo had worked hard to get ready for the race. Looking at their faces, I envied them.

What is it about the marathon? Is it the race's history? Its traditions? The many fine runners who have run it? The marathon is all of that, but there is also a mystique about the distance itself. Would the race have the same appeal if it were a more logical 25 miles, or 40 kilometers?

FOOTSTEPS OF PHEIDIPPIDES

The establishment of the marathon at the unquestionably odd distance of 26 miles 385 yards (or 42.2 kilometers) certainly adds to the mystique. The fact is that, technically speaking, *all* marathons are precisely 26 miles 385 yards. Anything longer and the race is considered an ultramarathon. Anything less and either the course was mismeasured or it is something else. The first event to be called a marathon was held in 1896 at the first modern Olympic Games in Athens, Greece. This long-distance footrace was staged at the end of those games to re-create and commemorate the legendary run of Pheidippides in 490 BC.

In that year, the Persians invaded Greece, landing near the plains of Marathon on Greece's eastern coast. Speaking at a pasta party the night before the 2010 Athens Marathon, Kathrine Switzer and Roger Robinson, co-authors of *26.2 Marathon Stories*, discussed the story that grew out of the Battle of Marathon 2,500 years before. According to legend, Miltiades, the victorious Athenian general, dispatched Pheidippides, a *hemerodromos*, or runner-messenger, to Sparta (150 miles away) to seek help. It reportedly took Pheidippides 2 days to reach Sparta. The Spartans never did arrive in time to help, but the Athenians eventually overwhelmed their enemy, killing 6,400 Persian troops while losing only 192 of their own men. Or so it was recorded by Greek historians of the time, including Herodotus, the most famous historian of the Classical Era of antiquity.

But was Pheidippides the same messenger who, according to legend, ran a route that took him south along the coast and up and across a series of coastal foothills before descending into Athens, a distance of about 25 miles from Marathon? He announced, "Rejoice! We conquer!" as he arrived in Athens—then fell over dead.

Ah, legends. Latter-day historians doubt the total accuracy of this legend. That includes Robinson and Switzer, who suggested at the pasta party that if there was a *hemerodromos*, he may not have been the same one known to have relayed the request for troops to Sparta. There may or may not have been a *hemerodromos* by the name of Pheidippides who died following a postbattle run to Athens. Robinson and Switzer note that Herodotus failed to mention a *hemerodromos*; the story appeared four centuries later, when the history of the battle was retold by Plutarch.

Every marathon ends in Athens.

Nevertheless, the co-authors concede: "Every marathon, somehow, ends in Athens." Speaking honestly, and maybe metaphorically, the legend took on the imprint of historical fact and was certainly no less worthy of respect than tales involving mythical Greek gods such as Hermes or Aphrodite, who supposedly emerged full-grown out of the brain of Zeus. It seemed perfectly reasonable at the 1896 Olympic Games to run a race in Pheidippides's honor from Marathon to the Olympic stadium in downtown Athens. It was particularly fitting that a Greek shepherd named Spiridon Loues won that event, the only gold medal in track and field won by the Greeks on their home turf.

Among the American clubs represented at those first Games was the BAA, whose team manager was John Graham. So impressed was Graham with this race that he decided to sponsor a similar event in his hometown the following year. Races of approximately 25 miles (40 kilometers) had taken place before in Europe, including one held in France before the Olympics. But nobody had attached the name *marathon* to these races, and there was not yet a marathon mystique.

Fifteen runners lined up at the start of the first Boston Athletic Association Marathon in 1897 to race from a side road in suburban Ashland into downtown Boston, and a legend was born. (A previous American marathon had been run in the fall of 1896 from Stamford, Connecticut, to Columbus Circle, near the finish line of the current New York City Marathon, but it failed to survive.) The Boston Marathon remains the oldest continuously held marathon. It has retained its status and prestige, and it attracted a record 35,868 finishers in 1996, its 100th running.

DETERMINING THE DISTANCE

For a dozen years, the official marathon distance was approximately 25 miles. That was the distance run in the 1900 Olympic Games in Paris and the 1904 Games in St. Louis, as well as in the Boston Marathon for its first twenty-eight years. Then, in 1908, in London, the British designed a marathon course that started at Windsor Castle and finished at the Olympic stadium. This was long before course certification experts measured race distances to an accuracy of plus or minus a few feet. Nobody challenged the British course design, which reportedly was laid out so that the royal family could see the start of the race. The distance from start to finish for that marathon was precisely 26 miles 385 yards. For whatever reason, that distance eventually became the standard for future marathons. The BAA waited until 1924 to lengthen its course, moving the starting line from Ashland to the nearby town of Hopkinton, where it is today.

Frank Shorter tells the story of running the marathon trials for the 1971 Pan American Games. At mile 21, he was in lockstep with Kenny Moore, a 1968 Olympian. "Why couldn't Pheidippides have died here?" Shorter groaned to Moore. In that case, it was Shorter who "died" and Moore who went on to win the race. Shorter one-upped Moore the following year at the Olympic Games in Munich, Germany, winning the gold medal, while Moore placed fourth and a third American, Jack Bachelor, placed ninth. That was the best showing by American marathoners in the Olympics until Meb Keflezighi and Deena Drossin (now Kastor) won silver and bronze medals, respectively, in Athens in 2004. In 2016 at the Olympic Games in Rio de Janeiro, Galen Rupp won the bronze medal.

The running event that is so popular today might not have been the same if the plain of Marathon had been closer to Athens. Exercise physiologists tell us that it is only after about 2 hours of running—or about 20 miles for an accomplished runner—that the body begins to fully deplete its stores of glycogen, the energy source that fuels the muscles. (Most half-marathoners do not hit the wall, because in going 13.1 miles, they probably do not completely deplete their glycogen stores.) Once glycogen is depleted, the body must rely more on fat, a less efficient fuel source. This is one of the reasons runners "hit the wall" at 20 miles. Successfully getting past that obstacle is what makes the marathon such a special event.

Twenty miles is the longest distance that I ask people using my training programs to run in practice for a marathon. I want runners—particularly those training for their first marathons—to touch the edge of the wall, not collide with it. You significantly increase your risk of injury and overtraining, both of which may negatively impact your race day performance, if you run much farther in practice. Many of us who consider ourselves accomplished runners run 20-milers as part of our marathon buildup without excessive pain and with little fanfare. It is only when we stretch beyond that point that people sit up and take notice. Would a million people line the roads along the Boston and New York City marathon routes if the distance were only 20 miles and there were no wall to conquer? No, they want to see us tempt the fate of Pheidippides. They come to see us suffer, although inevitably both spectator and runner leave fulfilled only if we demonstrate through our successful crashing through the wall and crossing of the finish line that we are victorious.

GLYCOGEN AND THE WALL

A term frequently used by marathoners is "hitting the wall." This usually occurs around 20 miles into the race, about the time the body runs out of energy. Often this happens so suddenly that runners feel as though they crashed into a brick wall. Their pace slows. Their breath becomes labored. They begin to walk. Finishing becomes a struggle. Then more of a struggle. It can be said that the first half of the marathon is 20 miles long; the second half, 6.2 more.

Physiologically, runners hit the wall when they deplete their muscles of glycogen. Glycogen is the sugarlike substance that serves as the main fuel for muscles during exercise. It is stored in the liver and muscles. When you run long distances, you deplete your glycogen stores and eventually run out of energy. With glycogen gone, the body begins burning fat, a much less efficient fuel source.

But not all runners hit the wall. With proper training, you can teach your body to burn fat more efficiently. Refueling on the run with sports drinks and gels adds to your glycogen supply. Proper pacing also will allow you to hurdle the feared wall and achieve a peak performance. I'm not kidding when I tell runners seeking last-minute advice at expos, "Start slow!"

CHANGING YOUR LIFE

For many runners, completing one marathon is enough. They cross the line and, overwhelmed with the experience, think, "Never again!" Only

13 miles into the Chicago Marathon and struggling, Nicole Kunz of McHenry, Illinois, swore to herself that she never—absolutely never—would run another marathon. Within 24 hours after finishing, however, Kunz already had begun to consider training for the Flying Pig Marathon in Cincinnati the following spring. She ran that marathon, then New York, before taking time off to have two children.

Kristine Nader of Chicago had a similar reaction during her first marathon: "I figured it would be one-and-done. The whole time I trained, I kept telling myself, 'This is nuts. Why am I doing this? What was I thinking? I am so glad I am only doing this once!'"

Then when she saw her family cheering her at mile 14, she realized this was something she wanted to do again—and again.

Marathoners may change their minds the next day, the next week, the next month, or sometimes as soon as they get to the end of the finish chute, but nobody can deny that a marathon—particularly a first marathon—is a very special event. A very, very special event. Finishing a marathon changes your life forever. Professional photographers who take pictures of runners crossing the finish line find marathoners make much better customers than those finishing shorter-distance events. Marathon photos outsell shorter-event photos by at least two to three times. People also buy multiple photos of themselves at the same marathon, compared with only a single photo at a shorter race. And among those who purchase one of my interactive training plans from TrainingPeaks, twice as many purchase full marathon plans as half marathon plans.

Why? It is for the same reason that people order more pictures at weddings. Completing a marathon is like tacking a PhD at the end of your name, getting married, or having a baby. You are special, and whether anyone else knows it or not, you certainly do. Your life will never again be quite the same, and regardless of what the future brings, you can look back and say, "I finished a marathon." Regardless of the large number of people running marathons today, you are still part of an elite crowd.

Some runners finish their first marathon, place their medal in a drawer, hang their photo on the wall of their office cubicle, and go on to different challenges. They can now check off another item on their bucket list. For many, however, that first marathon is merely the beginning of a lifetime journey. Running marathons becomes a continuing challenge of numbers: PRs, which exist to be broken at each race. Even when aging brings the inevitable decline in performance, new challenges arise as the lifetime marathoner moves from one five-year age bracket to another. In the area of performance, success breeds success.

It is also possible to run marathons recreationally, not caring about time or finishing position but participating merely for the joy of attending a great event with all its accompanying pleasures. I have run many marathons as a recreational tourist, running within myself and finishing far back from where I might have had I pushed the pace harder. One year at the Honolulu Marathon, I started in the back row and made a game out of passing as many people as possible—but doing it at a pace barely faster than theirs so as not to call attention to my speed. I did not want it to seem that I was trying to show them up. Beginning with the 1995 St. George (Utah)

> **Finishing a marathon changes your life forever.**

Marathon and prompted by an article I wrote ranking the marathon courses most likely to yield fast times so people could qualify for the 100th Boston Marathon, *Runner's World* began to organize pacing teams led by editors running slower than usual while shepherding others. It is fun and rewarding to help others meet their goals.

I have also run marathons in which I stopped at planned dropout points, using the race as a workout to prepare for later marathons. At the World Masters Track & Field Championships in Rome one year, I ran the marathon at the end of a week's track competition mainly so I could enjoy the sights and sounds of the Eternal City. In the last miles of the race, as I entered a piazza with a panoramic view of St. Peter's Cathedral across the Tiber River, I paused for several minutes to absorb that view before continuing toward the finish line in the stadium used for the 1960 Olympic Games. How fast I ran and how well I placed were the last things on my mind. Crossing the finish line, more refreshed than fatigued, I was approached by an Australian runner, who announced, "This is the first time I ever beat you."

I felt obliged to correct him: "You didn't beat me. You merely finished in front of me."

Okay, that was a bit rude, but the Australian had missed what I believed to be the point of that particular marathon. Or at least he was not aware of the way I had chosen to run the marathon that particular day. In a marathon, except at the elite level, you do not beat others, as you might in a 1-mile run or in a 100-meter dash. Instead, you achieve a personal victory. If others finish in front of or behind you, it is only that their personal victories are more or less than yours. A person finishing behind you with less talent or of a different age or sex or various other limiting factors may have achieved a far greater victory. And if the person's main goal in running the marathon was to raise money for charity, the amount collected may be a more important barometer of success than finishing time.

One beauty of the marathon is that there are many more winners than those who finish first overall or in their age groups. "Everyone's a winner" is a dreadful cliché, but it happens to be true when the race involved is 26 miles 385 yards long.

A LIFETIME OF MARATHONS

Over the years reporters and often other runners would ask how many marathons I had run. For many years, I would respond, "About a hundred."

This amazed them: "You've run a hundred marathons?"

I had to correct them because I did not want to read in the newspaper the next morning that I had just run marathon number 101. "No," I would say. "I don't know how many marathons I've run. But it must be about a hundred."

Then in the spring of 1995, a year before the 100th Boston Marathon, I got curious about the exact number. Using the BAA library, I searched through old running magazines and newsletters for past marathon results. I was able to identify several races that I had little memory of running, including one in which I had finished first! But the actual total number of marathons I had run was fewer than what I had been telling reporters for years: It was only ninety.

Yes, *only.*

That was the bad news, but the good news was that with a little effort over the next 12 months, I would be able to run my 100th marathon at the 100th Boston. Thus, running a marathon a month became my goal for a year.

Run ten more marathons I did, using the 100/100 challenge to motivate my training for more than a year—a very enjoyable year as I ran marathons from Memphis, Tennessee, to Hamilton, Bermuda, to Seaside, Oregon. That ninety-ninth marathon in Oregon, 1 month before the 100th Boston, fittingly was called the Trail's End Marathon, although Trail's Pause might have been a more appropriate name in my case, seeing as I still had to run the 100th Boston.

The 100th running of the Boston Marathon was one of the most difficult marathons of my career. That event coincided with the publication of *Boston: A Century of Running*, my coffee-table book published by Rodale commemorating the 100 years of the world's oldest running race. I spent most of the week before the race doing media interviews and then 3 days at the expo signing copies of the book and talking to runners—that plus a series of parties, including a Breakfast of Champions featuring most of those still living who had won the race. Amazingly, that included Canadian Johnny Miles, winner in 1926. It was a heady time, but by race day I was physically exhausted.

My wife, Rose, and I had rented a house on Hopkinton Common within sight of the starting line. Rather than line up with the masses that morning, I watched the start from the house's front yard, then went in to view the race on TV. The lead runners had passed 3 miles before Rose suggested, "Don't you think it's time to go run?"

I joined the runners in the back of the pack. The atmosphere seemed electric, every runner realizing that he or she was part of a truly historic occasion. But by 8 miles, my battery was fully discharged. I hit the wall well before there should have been any wall to hit. The Newton hills were still another 8 miles down course, but my previously steady stride had been reduced to a stumbling shuffle. And although it had seemed relatively warm in Hopkinton, with a tail wind pushing the runners, as we got closer to the ocean, the wind switched, becoming a chilling head wind. Near the halfway point, I picked up a discarded long-sleeved shirt from the gutter. It was soaked with sweat, but it helped keep me warm to near the top of Heartbreak Hill, where I spotted a Mylar space blanket, also discarded. I wrapped it around myself as one more defense against the cold wind off the ocean.

> **In the area of performance, success breeds success.**

I continued running and finished the 100th Boston in an unmemorable 6 hours, including the half hour or so it had taken me to cross the starting line after the gun sounded. (Chips that provide runners with the exact amount of time they spent between the starting line and finish line were not in general use at that time.)

One hundred being a round number, I probably should have called it a career, but I decided to lead pacing teams at the Chicago Marathon the next several years, then did the same at Honolulu. After running seven marathons in 7 months to celebrate my 70th birthday, I found myself with 111 marathons on my résumé: another number that sounded good when people asked how many I had run.

At an appearance at a running store in Kalamazoo, Michigan, one young woman who asked that question seemed amazed. "Eleven marathons?" she asked. "Wow, that's a lot."

"No, not eleven," I corrected her. "One hundred eleven marathons."

That truly dumbfounded the woman, but I am far from being the record holder when it comes to the number of marathons run. Sy Mah, a Toledo runner who often ran two and sometimes three marathons on a weekend, finished 524 races that were longer than 26 miles before his death from cancer at age 62 in 1988. Continually adding to the total was the focal point of Mah's running, so it was important that he kept precise records for each of his races. Mah usually finished in the high 3-hour range. I once told him that if he focused his attention for 6 months on a single race—training specifically for it, resisting the temptation to run other marathons so that he could taper and peak—he could probably improve his time by half an hour and maybe even break 3 hours, putting him near the top for his age group. Smiling, Sy conceded my point, but we both knew that was not what he was about. His joy was running as many marathons as possible and adding to his impressive string of numbers, which earned him an enviable spot in *The Guinness Book of World Records*. Incredibly, Sy amassed his total by taking time off winters, when he would enter cross-country ski races, such as the American Birkebeiner in Hayward, Wisconsin, 55 kilometers long. Since Sy's passing, other dedicated runners have surpassed his total, but he remains the ultimate champion to me. We all define our own goals.

The marathon never ceases to be a race of joy, a race of wonder. Even when disaster strikes, when bad weather overwhelms you, when an intemperate pace results in a staggering finish, when nerves and anxiety stand in the way of you giving your maximum effort, when your number one rival soundly thrashes you, when 18 weeks of training appear to have gone down the drain with little more than an ugly slurping sound, there remains something memorable about each marathon run.

The crying woman with whom I spoke before her first marathon in Chicago instinctively knew that fact. Her training leading up to that event certainly had been part of a lifetime change, a passage of sorts, one that sparked the flow of tears. If that becomes the only marathon she runs in a lifetime, it will be memorable. If she should continue to run additional marathons, each will be memorable, some more than others.

The marathon mystique continues to lure us to starting lines and finish lines. We are like moths drawn toward the flame.

YOUR FIRST MARATHON

Before starting to train for a marathon, you probably need to decide *which* marathon you want to run. Many factors can dictate your choice, one of them: Would you rather run a large marathon such as Chicago (44,610 finishers in 2018) or a relatively small race in the same state, the Illinois Marathon (1,140 finishers)? I posed this question on my Facebook page, and within 24 hours, nearly eight hundred respondents chose large marathon (69 percent) versus small marathon (31 percent). Their reasoning can guide you in picking your first 26-mile race.

Emma Friesen: If you're a back-of-the-packer, bigger events may be the only option to avoid running alone, or being asked to leave the course.

Amy Bannick Griffin: Large races always ensure you have fellow runners nearby. I hate being out there by myself.

Dave Schmidt: Small races have that friendly, hometown feel. The organizers make you feel like more than just a number on a bib.

Wayne Vn: Large races offer more support, and you are less likely to finish last. However unlikely, that is a big fear among many new runners.

Zsuzsanna Turanyi: Small. A lot smoother logistically. No need to get up so early. Easier parking. Less time standing on line. Fewer people slowing you down.

Reyna Merritt: Large. Good swag. Better support. Plenty of other runners out there with you so you don't feel alone or left behind.

Sydney Sorkin: Some find comfort in the energy of crowds, while others may like the peace of fewer people around them.

Many factors may determine which "first marathon" you decide to run. Select carefully, because it will be among the great experiences of your life.

2

Learning to Love Running

The Journey Is Part of the Reward

You can understand why new runners, first-timers, "newbies," as they sometimes are called, might approach the running of 26 miles 385 yards with a certain amount of fear. Seemed easy when you and your buddy double-dared each other at the bar last night, but now comes the hangover. Or maybe your decision to run a marathon comes from a promise made to join in lockstep with your girlfriend or boyfriend raising money for charity. People decide to run a marathon for various reasons.

But let's talk reality. How hard is it to train for a marathon? How difficult is it to push yourself out the door almost daily and run workouts up to 20 miles long? Could not somebody invent a pill that would produce instant fitness and allow us to complete races of 26 miles 385 yards without all that training, which must be both grueling and b-o-r-i-n-g, according to those who never have tried it?

Surprise! Most runners enjoy training for marathons. In a poll I took among participants in my Virtual Training Bulletin Boards, I discovered that three out of every four respondents liked training as much as or more than the marathon with all its pomp and splendor. The percentage of those who liked training best was 34 percent, versus 16 percent who enjoyed the marathon most. Thirty-nine percent claimed to like both equally.

So if you're starting one of my 18-week training programs and fear that running all that mileage may become a grind—particularly if your longest run up to now has been 2 or 3 miles—relax and enjoy. It may not seem so at the time, but looking back on your training after completing your first marathon, you may surprise yourself at how much fun it was, particularly if you trained with a like-minded group of individuals. Marathon running and the training leading up to it can be fun.

Typical of those responding to my survey was Lori Hauswirth from Merrill, Wisconsin. "The marathon is the reward, and the training is actually the harder of the two," claims Hauswirth. "But they are both equally enjoyable. Training does absorb a lot of time, but few everyday people can say they've ever been as dedicated to anything as those of us who train 18 weeks for a marathon."

> **Marathon running and the training leading up to it can be fun.**

Christine Zelenak, of Alexandria, Virginia, concurs. "Although I thoroughly enjoyed my first marathon, the training leading up to it was the most empowering thing I had ever done, at least physically," Zelenak says. "Every week was a highlight, with a new distance record set. I had that same excitement at mile 20 of the marathon, when I knew I was really going to finish it. But it was the journey that transformed me. The marathon was the reward."

John Grasser of Chevy Chase, Maryland, says, "Immediately after my first marathon, I reflected on the previous 18 weeks and realized that while the race itself was the reward, it was really all that training over the months that made it fun and all worth it. I realized how much I looked forward to those long Sunday runs. And all that training put me in the best shape of my life. I was able to say I had accomplished something not many others had, having run 26.2 miles."

"The marathon is the destination," adds Martin Conlon from Wheeling, Illinois, "but getting there is what it's all about."

THE CHALLENGE

Jim Fredericks of South Milwaukee, Wisconsin, has run frequent marathons and has experienced often the cycle of train-race-relax. Fredericks looks forward to the challenge of each new week as the long runs keep getting longer and longer—and longer. "I count the runs and count the days," he says. "I am very aware of the surroundings on my running trail and watch as the environment goes from late spring through the summer and into early autumn. Working toward achieving a personal goal is fun and rewarding. The race itself is such a great experience. The atmosphere in the host city can be invigorating. I think training and the race are equally rewarding. I start to plan my next race and training cycle almost as soon as I am finished with the last one."

"The marathon provides a goal, an incentive, and a focus," says Autumn Evans from Melbourne Beach, Florida. "Without the marathon, there is less reason to get out and train hard. Yes, one should exercise for one's health, but good health often is taken for granted; thus, we don't always do what we know we should.

"I was able to say I had accomplished something."

"Completing a marathon, however, provides material rewards: a shirt, a medal, a certificate, and one's name in lights—or at least in the results booklet. In addition to the tangible benefits, the race itself offers entertainment, starting with the expo and ending with the finish line festivities. There's a feeling of camaraderie in the back of the pack that isn't present in many sports. Runners take care of each other, encourage each other, push each other. It's competition, but competition with oneself. Imaginative spectators post signs that bring smiles to the faces of weary runners. Venturesome athletes run in hilarious costumes. And before and during and after the event, race shirts or limping gaits or overheard discussions cause total strangers to strike up conversations."

Though she has completed dozens of marathons, Melissa Vetricek from Tampa, Florida, has only begun to understand the event. "I'm still learning," she says, "but I consider the marathon itself more enjoyable than the training. Some training runs are fun, but other training runs— let's be honest—are not fun. You struggle through them because you see the carrot dangling before your eyes. The marathon is something I look forward to with eager anticipation and with each training run. It's hard not to when each run has a specific distance and effort level all with the purpose of preparing me to cover 26.2 miles as quickly as I can on race day. I guess I'm just such a goal-oriented person that only after I reach the goal am I able to relax and enjoy what I accomplished. Then it's time to set a new goal all over again!"

> **"It was the journey that transformed me. The marathon was the reward."**

Cindy Southgate of Kanata, Ontario, uses visual goals to motivate herself as she trains. "I love watching the days go by," says Southgate. "I have my schedule printed out and highlight each workout as it is completed. There's a great sense of accomplishment seeing the weeks go by, as well as watching my progress."

Dave Dwyer from Madison, Wisconsin, says: "It is hard to beat the excitement, the actual physical thrill, the relief and joy and pride, when you see the finish line in your first marathon and can say, 'I'm a marathoner.' It is hard to beat the anticipation of the night before, the jumble of pleasure the morning of the event, and the thrill that rolls down your spine when you hear the starting gun. People haven't even begun to move forward and already they're crying.

"The run itself kind of melts along with the other training runs, which have their moments, too. It is a journey, a long distance of revelation of self, of accomplishment and of failure, of goals met and those still ahead.

After all of that, the medal is only icing on the cake. It is the inner warmth of the accomplishment that remains with you, medal or not."

"I like training and the marathon itself for what they bring to my life," says Chicagoan Randy Egge. "The training lasts months and is part of my routine and lifestyle. The training is the main course. When the race comes around, I am almost sad because it signifies that part of my daily routine, which I love, will be gone for a while. I look at the race like I look at dessert at the end of a fine meal."

"If I didn't enjoy the training, I would never run marathons," says Liz Reichman from San Antonio, Texas.

"Through the training, you learn so much about your limits physically and mentally as a runner," says Chicagoan Lisa Schumacher. "The process is fun, because you discover that you can overcome obstacles and become a better runner. What you believe in your mind is what your body will do. Training for the marathon distance forces that out of you."

> **Runners take care of each other, encourage each other, push each other.**

"I like the training a lot more than the marathon itself," says Amber Balbier of Dallas, Texas. "I just plain love to run, and I'm happiest when my training is at its peak. I enjoy the spice that the advanced training plans have to offer, incorporating different types of running. Tapering, nerves, nutrition, and the stress of the marathon make me crazy. One wrong move, bad day, or bad weather and the time goal is out the window.

"All that said, the mystique of the marathon keeps me coming back for more. Marathoning is an art as much as a science, and I look forward to the day when everything comes together and I achieve the pitch-perfect performance. I live for that day."

"I like the buildup during training," says New Yorker Dave Wolfe, "looking back at the log and seeing how the little weekly advances result in increased fitness. Even after a bad marathon, there is nothing better than knowing you put in the time and training to give it your best effort on a given day."

Seth Harrison, also a New Yorker, claims, "While running marathons is my ultimate reward for all the training, there's nothing quite like structuring 18 weeks of my life around a marathon training cycle. There's an electricity that I can't quite put my finger on that I feel during those weeks; and as I check off each daily workout and then each week of the training cycle, the anticipation and that electricity build and build. Nothing compares to standing at the starting line, then using all that training for its intended purpose, and ultimately crossing the finishing line with a sense of accomplishment that defies words."

> **"Marathoning is an art as much as a science."**

Finally, consider the words of Peg Coover from Cairo, Nebraska: "The satisfaction when it is over and I have finished another 26.2 is amazing!"

That is the lure that attracts all of us to the marathon.

MARATHON # 1

In a marathon with fifty thousand runners, there certainly must exist fifty thousand stories. Several of my friends on Facebook recall how they felt about Marathon #1.

Frank Tiburzi, Jr., started running late in life, after a bout of cancer. "I ran a 5K as a survivor," says Tiburzi. "That first 5K led to a 10K to a half and finally my first full marathon at age 56."

Shannon Lea chose Grandma's Marathon in Duluth, Minnesota, for her first marathon. "I loved the training and every minute of the race. I signed up for my next marathon almost immediately, that time running for charity."

(continued)

Kim Thayer ran the Portland Marathon and after crossing the finish line knew she was hooked. "I set a goal then to run Boston. It took me 6 years to achieve that goal, but running the Boston Marathon was a dream come true."

Emily Deutsch chose Sioux Falls, South Dakota, but on an unbearably hot and humid day. "I watched a woman dry heave at mile 5 and a man get whisked away in an ambulance halfway. I didn't know what I was getting myself into, but I finished."

Francisco Ortiz ran his first marathon in Dallas. "I hit the wall hard at 20 and limped to a 4:00 finish. I didn't run another for three years, but with better training, I knocked a half hour off my time."

Brian W. Snyder did his first marathon in Pittsburgh after turning 40: "Crossing the finish line in my first felt like one of the greatest accomplishments in my life. I've run three more marathons since."

Darren James struggled during his first marathon in Dublin, Ireland. "The pain was unreal. I thought, 'Never again.' The following year I entered Dublin again, and my most recent 26-miler was Berlin."

Dominique Gallant after running Chicago thought, "I am numb. I can't walk. This was the hardest thing I have ever done. I want to do another."

Troy Miller claims that he was out of it after he crossed the finish line of his first marathon, in Olathe, Kansas. "And even while I was out of it, I still remember thinking, 'I actually did it!'"

Leanne Loney was happy to be done after number one. "My feet felt like they were wood blocks, but the feeling of accomplishment was intense." She ran marathons 14, 15, 16, and 17 in Vancouver, Quebec, Berlin, and Chicago.

Stephanie Churchill ran her first marathon in Baltimore. "It was so much fun I immediately knew I wanted to do many more."

Judy Loy did her first one in 1983. "I thought it would be the only one, but I loved it so much that I've done 67 more (including a few 50Ks). Four more planned for this year."

Gonzalo Quintana picked Madrid for number one. "I had a lot of respect for the distance, so I ran very carefully. Since then I have completed another 23 all over Europe. The marathon will continue with me until the end of my days."

3

Your First Steps

Take Those First Few Steps Cautiously

What is the minimum level of fitness needed for someone to begin training for a marathon? I once thought I knew the answer, although I'm less cocksure now. In the introduction to my 18-week Novice 1 training program, I once offered this answer to that question.

> People differ greatly in ability, but ideally before starting a marathon program, you should have been running about a year. You should be able to run distances between 3 and 6 miles. You should be training 3 to 5 days a week, averaging 15 to 25 miles a week. You should have run an occasional 5K or 10K race. It is possible to run a marathon with less of a training base (particularly if you come from another sport), but the higher your fitness level, the easier this 18-week program will be.

I still believe in those guidelines—particularly the final comment, that the higher your fitness level at the start of marathon training, the easier it will be to continue and complete that training—but I have come to modify my opinion of who should and who should not start training for a marathon. That's because I've seen too many people with a lesser training base suddenly decide, almost on a whim, to run a marathon—and they have succeeded!

Not everyone should approach a marathon lightly, but if you are young and highly motivated (and maybe just a little foolish) or suddenly decide you want to join a friend or complete a marathon to raise money for a charity, let me help.

How much base training do most new runners have? In one survey I conducted, 41 percent said that they had been running at least a year before they ran their first marathon. Another 28 percent had done some training before committing to one of my 18-week programs. Thus, at least two out of every three new marathoners had done *some* base training before committing to an 18-week training program like mine. Nevertheless, not everyone arrives well prepared. One individual queried me on-

> **"Every time I wanted to smoke, I ran instead."**

line 3 weeks before a marathon, wondering if it was too late to start! Everybody told him to wait until next year. We never did find out whether he heeded our advice or, if not, how he fared in the marathon with so little preparation.

Still, some people jump off the diving board without bothering to determine how deep the water is below. A friend of mine—Bill Wenmark from Minnetonka, Minnesota—admitted to running his first marathon with that little training: 3 weeks and a total of 23 miles running! A former hockey player, Bill figured he could pass the test without studying or doing homework. Wenmark finished in just under 6 hours, but he had so trashed his leg muscles that it forced him to drive his Volkswagen stick-shift car home without using the clutch. Pushing the pedal hurt too much. Bill learned from his mistakes, eventually lowered his marathon time to under 3 hours, and has now coached four thousand new runners to do the opposite of what he did.

I didn't design my online training program guidelines to discourage people. I was just being realistic about what it takes to finish a marathon comfortably. Indeed, some people responding to my survey said they were encouraged by my guidelines. For example, Bill Rieske of Orem, Utah, wrote: "I was thinking a marathon was out of reach until I read your guidelines. The part that made me attempt one was 'It is possible to run a marathon with less of a training base.' I had run a 5K and 10K but wasn't averaging anything near 15 to 25 miles a week. Everything else I had read warned: 'Don't do a marathon until you've been running a year.' I trained as best as I could and slowly gained confidence that I could finish. I did that but realized how much easier it would have been with a better training base. I built on that base leading up to my second marathon and finished feeling more comfortable." Rieske ran his first marathon in 4:15 and his second in 3:35 on the same course.

"I had run on and off before training for a marathon," comments Liz Reichman of San Antonio, Texas. "I was generally active, doing spinning, stair-climbing, weight lifting, even aerobics, but not running. I approached the training knowing I was in great shape but not great running shape." Reichman ran 4:14 in her first marathon. She eventually would drop her PR to 3:57 and run forty marathons.

Reno, Nevada, resident David McGraw had been a high school athlete who biked and skied to stay in shape. Then he decided to run a marathon. McGraw jogged for 3 months before starting a structured training program. Despite this background, he found running the marathon to be "a lesson in pain and humility."

Carleen Pruess Coulter from Shorewood, Illinois, started running in her midtwenties to help her stop smoking: "Every time I wanted to smoke, I ran instead." After 3 months, she started training for a marathon. Reflecting on that event 2 decades later, Coulter admits, "I probably should not have rushed into a marathon, because the race was very hard for me, but it kept me from smoking and was worth it."

LEARNING TO RUN

Runners arrive at the starting line of a marathon with varying degrees of ability and experience. In a related survey, I asked how many people had run the marathon as their first race of any distance. Based on conversations with many new runners, I expected that a large percentage would tell me that the marathon, indeed, was their first running race. But only 15 percent reported that to be true. Among those who had raced shorter distances, the half marathon was the most popular first-race choice (20 percent).

When I first put my marathon training programs online, I actually discouraged first-timers from doing any other races, which I considered a diversion. Since then, I have begun singing a new tune, now recommending that newcomers run at least one or two races to get a feel for what it is like to go to a starting line. The half marathon is also a handy distance for predicting performance in the marathon to come.

Charles Romano from Maplewood, New Jersey, followed the half marathon route. "My first race was a half, which I used as a goal to keep motivated," says Romano. "By the time I achieved that goal, I realized I enjoyed running. My second race was a marathon later that same year."

Judging from my surveys, I can see that the individual who has never taken a running step before committing to a first marathon may not exist—or exists only as an anomaly. Even though individuals may not consider themselves "runners," they often have participated in other activities that provided at least some base of fitness before they began.

Running is a basic activity, instinctive to our being. People need not be taught how to run. Children learn to run almost as soon as they learn to walk. Visit any elementary school playground and you will see kids sprinting all over the place. All children are born sprinters.

Children modify their behavior as they get older. Running starts to become a discipline rather than a natural form of exercise. An athlete who goes out for any sport in high school—football, basketball, tennis, whatever—runs as part of the conditioning for that sport. High school athletes run either because their coach tells them to or because they know that getting in shape will help them make the team. Or sometimes if they miss a free throw or drop a pass, they are forced to run a lap around the field. (I love the T-shirt seen sometimes at cross-country races: "My sport is your sport's punishment.") Usually, young athletes run what in the track world might be called a middle distance: a few laps on a track, then off to the main activity. It is only as adults that people forget how to run and sometimes need to be retaught.

So let us talk about being a beginning runner. Before you can hope to cover long distances, you must start by running short distances—and running them slowly. Some beginners (particularly if they're overweight) need to walk first, beginning with half an hour 3 or 4 days a week. Then they start to jog a short distance until they get slightly out of breath, walk to recover, jog some more. Jog, walk. Jog, walk. Jog, walk. After a while, they will be able to run a mile without stopping.

> **Running is a basic activity, instinctive to our being.**

Before we move forward, some important kernels of information are hidden in what I have just said. Even experienced runners can learn from it.

The pattern is this: Jog, walk. Jog, walk. Jog, walk. Expressed another way: Hard, easy. Hard, easy. Hard, easy. The most effective training programs—even at the basic level—mix bursts of difficult running with rest. Train, rest. Train, rest. Train, rest.

Rest! That may be the most important word you will read in this book. (You'll encounter it again and again.) In the questionnaire I sent to coaches to gather information for the first edition of this book, one of the questions was: "How important is rest in the training equation?"

The first coach to return a completed questionnaire was Paul Goss of Foster City, California. His response was simple and direct: "More important than most runners know."

None of the other coaches who eventually responded improved on what Goss had to say.

GET OFF THE COUCH

With beginners, the problem is not to get them to rest but to get them to stop resting. Couch potatoes need to get off the couch and away from the TV. They need to learn to become participants in sport rather than spectators of sport. To those of us who accept running as a natural activity, the shift from spectator to participant is not as easy as it may seem.

Beginners need motivation to begin—and to keep at it once they have begun. "The key factor in any beginner's training program is motivation," suggests Jack Daniels, PhD, an exercise physiologist and former coach at the State University of New York College at Cortland. "If you're genetically gifted but not interested in training, you'll never develop."

Barring some medical problem, most people can run, but they are not motivated to do so. Even if they want to start running, it takes courage to put on running shoes and step out on a sidewalk for the first time in front of friends and neighbors. A lot of potential runners never get moving, out of fear of looking foolish. They lack self-confidence. They fear failure.

It sometimes helps to join a class. Many running clubs offer classes for beginning runners. One advantage of a class situation is the group support you get from others of equal ability (or lack of ability). The most important information any coach can offer beginners is not how to hold their arms or how far to jog without stopping but simply this: "You're looking good. You're doing great. Keep it up." Basic motivation. Once you start, natural running instincts, overlooked but not forgotten from childhood, will take over.

Joining a beginner's running program can provide you with support, information, and good training routes, but in particular it can give you motivation as you train with others. If you are looking for a program in your area, check with local health clubs, running clubs, specialty running stores, or the organizers of major races. One good source of information is the Road Runners Club of America (RRCA), which has nearly one thousand member clubs, with two hundred thousand individual runners. The RRCA has trained more than six thousand certified adult running coaches. (You can find an RRCA Certified Coach in every state.) The organization's website (rrca.org) lists clubs and contact information.

TrainingPeaks, the endurance training platform and organization that hosts my interactive training programs, also has a stable of twelve thousand coaches, who work with runners as well as swimmers, cyclists, and triathletes. You can search the TrainingPeaks Coach Directory to get matched with an accredited coach using their Coach Match Service. Although at various times in my career, I have coached individuals, sports teams, and adult classes, I now limit my coaching to those who follow me online. Thus, I serve as a vehicle to the good coaching that exists if you search for it.

And the beat goes on. After graduating from the University of Notre Dame, where he competed in track and cross-country, my grandson Kyle Higdon coached students at the University of Texas at Austin while studying for a PhD in aeronautical engineering. Now working for NASA in Houston, Kyle has begun to coach runners in that organization not for pay but because he enjoys doing it.

We are drawn to the marathon, but before beginning to think about running, much less running such a stressful race, there are some precautions you need to take.

LEARN TO LOVE STRESS

People older than age 35 who want to start exercising should consider having a medical examination, including possibly an exercise stress test. The ACSM recommends testing at age 40 for men and age 50 for women—if you're apparently healthy. But if you have any risk factors for coronary artery disease (high blood pressure, high cholesterol, smoking, diabetes, or a family history of heart problems), you should be tested prior to vigorous exercise at any age.

The cardiology departments of many major medical centers provide exercise stress tests for $750 to $1,000—expensive, but your insurance policy may reduce the charges to near zero. Or you may be able to get the test done in a physician's office for as little as $150, says one hospital director. The best type of test is "symptom limited," in which you exercise until you attain your maximum tolerated exercise workload. If symptoms develop, the cardiologist may stop the test, but Paul D. Thompson, MD, director of preventive cardiology at Hartford Hospital in Connecticut, suggests that you avoid letting the cardiologist stop you when you reach your age-predicted maximum heart rate. "This 'maximum heart rate' varies a lot among individuals," says Dr. Thompson. "Using it as a stopping point can deny you a true maximal test."

With beginners, the problem is not to get them to rest but to get them to stop resting.

In a stress test, a cardiologist uses an electrocardiograph (EKG) to monitor your heartbeat while you walk or jog on a treadmill. Or you may be tested as you pedal an ergometer (exercise bicycle). The cardiologist will also record blood pressure. If your coronary arteries are even partially blocked, it should become apparent during stress. Changes in your heartbeat will appear on the EKG screen, and you will be asked to stop. This does not mean you cannot run, but you will need to begin under careful medical supervision. Doctors regularly prescribe exercise, including running, for patients who have had heart attacks. It is not uncommon for people with a history of heart issues, even those who have had quadruple bypass operations, to finish marathons.

But if this is you, don't do it alone. Seek supervision and support to make certain you can run 26.2 miles safely.

I have had numerous stress tests during a long running career, several of them supervised by *Aerobics* author Dr. Ken Cooper at his Cooper

Clinic in Dallas. While doing research for various magazine articles and books, I have watched others being tested. Most memorable was at a lab in Oslo, Norway, where the runner pushed so hard toward the end to reach the highest possible VO_2 max (the maximum amount of oxygen the body can utilize during a specified period of exercise) that he flew off the end of the moving belt and into the wall. Apparently, he was not the only Norwegian runner to do just that, because the walls surrounding the treadmill were heavily padded.

I don't suggest that others push that hard, particularly not beginners. If no symptoms develop during your exam—and assuming there are no other medical problems—you will be cleared to start running.

Just because you pass an exercise stress test once, however, is no guarantee you will never have a heart attack, either while running or while engaged in other activities. Physicians now recommend that you have a physical every two to three years, more often as you get older or if your cardiologist determines you're in a high-risk category. Also, learn the heart attack symptoms. The classic signs include chest pain but can include any generalized pain between the eyeballs and the belly button, even a toothache; often, a woman will feel nausea and fatigue. Their symptoms often differ from those of men. If such symptoms develop during a run, stop immediately and seek medical advice. Even if the symptoms seem to diminish as you continue to run, that does not mean that you are safe.

HOW TO BEGIN

My apologies to experienced runners who have been there, done that, but everybody has to begin somewhere. First, put on a pair of comfortable shoes. Although you will eventually need shoes specifically designed for running, for your first couple of short outings, you can wear whatever sports shoe you have.

Start to jog gently, on a smooth or soft surface, Have a hard time covering even 100 yards? Don't be discouraged. It is a beginning. If possible, jog until you are somewhat out of breath, then begin to walk. Resume jogging when you feel comfortable, walking again if necessary. When your tired muscles will not let you jog any farther, finish by walking.

If you never have run before, focus your attention on time rather than distance or pace. Set as your goal 30 minutes of combined jogging and walking. Start by walking for 10 minutes: no running allowed. For the next 15 minutes, you are free to run or walk. Then finish the workout with 5 minutes of walking. This is my 30/30 plan, featuring 30 minutes a day for 30 days. If you need more rest, consider my 30/60 plan, training every other day—thus, 60 days.

Record your time in a diary, on a calendar, or in an online training log. Do not worry about distance and pace this early in your training.

WHEN TO RUN

Run at a time that is convenient for you. Here are the advantages and disadvantages of running at different times of the day:

Morning. Many, if not most, runners run in the morning, before they eat breakfast. It is a good way to begin the day. Running can both wake you up and refresh you. If you run in the dark (common in winter), wear a reflective vest so motorists can see you. The one downside of training at this hour is that morning runners seem to get injured more often than afternoon runners. That's probably because they are stiff after just getting out of bed. To combat this problem, start your morning run by walking or running very slowly, then stop to do some brief stretching exercises before continuing.

Midday. If you have an hour or more for lunch, you may be able to squeeze in a workout at this time. Some offices have health clubs with showers and encourage workers to exercise at midday. Learn to manage your time. Plan your lunch in advance so you

(continued)

can grab a quick cup of yogurt or bowl of soup before returning to work. Noon, when temperatures are usually warmer, is a good time to run during the winter, but for that same reason it's a bad time during the dog days of summer.

Evening. Stop for a workout on your way home from work. Or go for a quick run after returning home and before dinner. This may not work if you are the one who is expected to put food on the table or have kids waiting to be fed. If this is the case, negotiate days when you and your spouse can alternate training and homemaking. Late evening, after the kids go to bed, is another option, but this probably means running in the dark. *You should always run in a safe area.* There are some places where you do not want to run alone, even in the daytime.

Weekend. On Saturdays and Sundays, most runners have more time for training. That being the case, you may want to plan your workout week so that you do most of your mileage on the weekends. Most runners (particularly those training for a marathon) do their long runs on the weekend.

Anytime. Who says you need to run at the same time every day? There is a virtue in regularity, but you can also get caught in a rut. Once running becomes a regular part of your lifestyle, feel free to experiment with different training patterns.

If you chose the easier 30/60 approach, take the next day off. On the third day, repeat the first day's workout, but again, do not worry about distance. If you go much farther or faster than the first day, you may be progressing too rapidly. Take the fourth day off.

On the fifth day, again repeat the basic workout, then rest the sixth day. Your training has followed the classic hard/easy pattern used by former University of Oregon track coach Bill Bowerman and countless other top coaches in training world-class runners. The pattern is the same; only the degree of difficulty is different.

The second week, simply repeat the workouts you did during the first week. You may feel that you can run farther or go faster, but hold back. When Bowerman developed his championship athletes at the University of Oregon, he always felt it was better that they be somewhat undertrained than overtrained. Even though there was a chance the Oregon athletes might perform slightly below their potential while undertrained, their chances for injury were greatly reduced. If that conservative approach made sense for his highly talented athletes, members of numerous Olympic teams, why shouldn't it also work for you?

Almost all training designed to improve runners is based on advancing from level to level.

The second week is critical in any beginning running program. You may have been able to run through Week 1 just from sheer beginner's enthusiasm, but now you are into Week 2. Your muscles are sore, you are getting bored with the same every-other-day routine, and it has dawned on you that you probably will never win an Olympic gold medal. And it may feel as if running will never get any better.

Hang in there. It will.

CONTINUING TO RUN

How fast should you be running? It doesn't matter. Again, you should be worrying about time, not distance or pace. You can record distance and pace, but if you try to increase either, you are more likely to get injured. Better to go too slow in the beginning than too fast.

Remember that bit of advice I offered to runners who approached me at expos the day before their marathon: *Start slow!*

Almost all training designed to improve runners is based on advancing from level to level. You work harder and improve, moving from a low level to a higher level. This is your body's progressive adaptation to increasing stress. My 18-week marathon training programs, which you will encounter later in the book, feature increases of approximately 1 mile a week for the weekend long runs. Over that 18-week time period, weekly mileage doubles. The changes in numbers are small; the changes in fitness and the body's capacity to adapt to stress are great.

Later in this book, I offer marathon training programs for novice, intermediate, and advanced runners, with two separate programs at each level. Not everybody can move from the first level in training to the second and then to the third. If you overtrain, you are likely to crash. Even if you do not injure yourself, you may discover that your competitive efforts deteriorate. You begin to run slower instead of faster. Sooner or later, this happens to almost all top athletes.

Elite athletes are constantly pushing the envelope, trying to measure the limits of human performance. There are two ways to learn about training. One is by having access to a knowledgeable coach; the other is by trial and error. With a knowledgeable coach, you make training errors less frequently.

MAXIMIZING PERFORMANCE

How can you maximize your performance? How much can you improve? When asked how much improvement runners might expect by following a year's hard training, Dr. Jack Daniels, the exercise physiologist and well-known coach, initially suggested 5 percent as an upper limit. But it is a tough question. "There is no physiological basis for saying how much you can increase your workload," he finally admitted. Runners differ enormously in both their capabilities and their capacities, he says: "Some people with little training background have tremendous potential for improvement. Others who have been running for many years may have improved as much as they can."

Let me add one more key word that determines whether you can maximize performance: motivation. Without the motivation to begin, without the motivation to continue, you ain't getting very far. "The miracle is not that I finished," *Runner's World* contributor John Bingham used to say. "The miracle is that I had the courage to start."

Every beginner will improve with practice. Here are four areas in which runners can improve in ability.

1. **Oxygen delivery:** Strengthen the heart muscle and your oxygen delivery system becomes more efficient.
2. **Oxygen absorption:** As you train, you also will increase blood flow through the muscle fibers and at the same time strengthen those fibers. This improves the body's ability to use oxygen.
3. **Economy:** As you continue to run, your technique and form will improve, allowing you to expend energy more efficiently.
4. **Endurance:** You can run farther and faster before hitting your pain threshold. Stronger muscles contract more effectively.

To improve to the highest level requires talent. But even people of average talent can rise above their abilities and achieve extremely high levels of success as runners. In perhaps no event is this truer than in the marathon.

4

Beginnings

The First Time Is Always Very Special

Michael Young vividly remembers his first marathon. A resident of Orchard Lake, Michigan, Young had run in high school but never a marathon. He recalls: "Even back then, Boston was in the back of my mind, as though on some sort of bucket list."

But by age 50, Young still had not run any marathon, much less Boston. Then his father died of complications from Parkinson's disease. The last of Young's six children was only four. "I decided then it was important that I last long enough to see my youngest at least finish college," he says. "I figured getting in better shape would be a good first step."

Young began running around the neighborhood, eventually working up to four miles. Two of his sisters had been All-American swimmers as well as runners. They suggested that to stay motivated, he target some race. Young chose the Detroit Turkey Trot, a Thanksgiving 10K with eighteen thousand runners. "I barely broke 50 minutes," he remembers, "but I felt like the local champion!" Next, his sisters (both Boston qualifiers) suggested they run a marathon together, choosing the Marine Corps Marathon in Washington, D.C., the following fall. (Young's third sister lived in D.C.) For several months he resisted, but he finally registered in April. This convinced his brother and their nonrunning sister to join what had become a family fun run. "Now we had all five siblings running," he says. "We recruited a friend and a brother-in-law, and then we had seven."

Unfortunately, Young's mother passed away only a year after his father died. "We ran the marathon in honor of our parents, five of the seven of us achieving Boston qualifiers and the other two going the distance," Young says. "We all achieved our objective."

People decide to run marathons for varying reasons. Koen van Urk of the Netherlands claims that he first ran a marathon after a bet with his boss. In a poll on Twitter, many runners told me they moved up to the 26.2-mile distance as the logical step after several years, or even several decades, of running shorter distances. Others chose the marathon as the ultimate challenge: "If I can do this, I can do almost anything!" Or they became inspired by others they knew who ran. The desire to improve health lures many to the starting line. So does weight loss.

Finishing should be your first goal, maybe your only goal.

Scott Kalina from Palatine, Illinois, started running to improve his health and lose a few pounds. "One October, I went into the city to see what the Chicago Marathon was all about," he says. "I missed the start but went to several locations to watch runners stream by. Later I stood at the finish line for at least 45 minutes, watching the joy and pain of the finishers between 3 and 4 hours." Kalina stopped at a bookstore and purchased a copy of this book. The following October he was among the Chicago finishers, running 5 hours, eventually improving to 4:37.

A few runners accept the challenge to prove something, both to themselves and to their friends. Bob Winter from New Lenox, Illinois, ran his first marathon because his friends doubted he could do even one. "That became a huge motivator for me on those days when I didn't want to go out and run," Winter recalls. "After that, I was hooked, and now I do marathons because I love setting goals and working hard to reach them."

Though a runner for many years, Seth Harrison considered the marathon distance out of his reach. "Most years," Harrison recalls, "I would cover the finish of the New York City Marathon and photograph the winners. These world-class elites seemed like in a different universe. I never considered what they were doing as being the same as the type of running I did. Then one year, I stayed long enough to see the 4- and 5-hour runners crossing the finish line with hands raised over their heads like they had just won the race. That was it for me." Six months later, Harrison ran the Pocono Marathon, finishing in 3:41.

Seattle's Starrla Johnson ran track and cross-country in high school but never considered running a marathon until she visited a friend who worked at a hotel near the finish line of the Boston Marathon. Johnson recalls: "On the day of the marathon, I sat on a newspaper box for 3 hours, totally entranced, watching runners stream across a yellow line painted on the street. I laced up my running shoes that evening. My first run took me 2 miles."

A year and a half later, Johnson finished her first marathon, running 4:05 at the Baystate Marathon in Lowell, Massachusetts. "I loved calling my high school coach and telling him I just ran a marathon," says Johnson. "I loved even more calling him three marathons later and telling him I qualified for Boston."

THE THREE GOALS

Once you decide to run that first marathon, there are three goals worth considering: (1) to finish, (2) to improve, and (3) to win. Which goal you strive for depends on your level of running, and what you bring to the training table.

1. TO FINISH

To finish is important to the beginning or novice marathoner. To paraphrase Vince Lombardi: Finishing isn't everything; it's the only thing. More and more runners are running their first marathons these days. At some marathons, nearly 40 percent of the field may consist of first-timers. For them, covering 26 miles 385 yards equals victory. The fact that the marathon creates so many winners is one of its appeals.

Regardless of time, regardless of place, the primary goal is to get to the finish line standing up and in reasonably good shape. Friends and relatives do not want to hear about your time—they just want to hear that you finished. Finishing should be your first goal, maybe your only goal. Finish with a smile on your face. Finish knowing you might have done better if you had trained a bit harder or pushed the pace earlier. Run and train conservatively for your first marathon.

Time goals are important only for experienced runners. Worry about your time only if you run a second or third marathon. Set as your primary first-marathon goal enjoying the experience. Regardless of how fast or slow you run—unless you set your goal too high—you will look back on that first completed marathon as a significant experience, a momentous occasion in your life.

Whether you enjoy the experience as a first-time marathoner enough to become a next-time marathoner may be irrelevant. For most beginners, to finish is to win. And for many, once is enough.

2. TO IMPROVE

To improve is the goal of the seasoned runner. "Seasoned" could describe anybody who has run for several years, who has finished a first marathon—or two or three—and wants to run faster. For these runners, improving from 6 hours to 5, from 5 hours to 4, from 4 hours to 3, or various gradients within those hour blocks is akin to victory. Setting personal records is the name of the game for many of us. It doesn't matter if the PR is for your career, your current age group, the year, or the month of June. Take your victories where you can find them.

Improvement does not come easily. You have to work at it. On my website and in this book, I offer nearly a dozen marathon training programs for runners at various levels: novice, intermediate, and advanced. Each program provides a slight step up in difficulty. If you finished your first one or two marathons by following my Novice 1 or Novice 2 schedules, you may need to move to Intermediate 1 or Intermediate 2, featuring increased mileage, in order to improve in future marathons. Eventually, you may decide to take the final step up to Advanced 1 or Advanced 2, adding speedwork and other means of fine-tuning your skills (or compensating for lack of skills). You may need to add supplemental exercises, lift weights, and learn to stretch properly and eat right to get better. You may even want to hire a coach, one who works one-on-one with you, telling when to train harder and when to back off.

> **Set as your primary first-marathon goal enjoying the experience.**

If you run many marathons, at some point in your life it becomes increasingly difficult to snip seconds off your PR. And inevitably, if you stay in marathoning long enough, improvement may become impossible—at least as measured on the clock.

Nevertheless, each move to a new age group (five years) provides an opportunity for improvement within that group. And as an aging runner's career ascends peaks and drops into valleys, it becomes possible to allow yourself to sink to new lows by backing off training so that you can establish new highs by increasing that training. For some runners, every marathon is like their first; each one is a new adventure. Even after 111 marathons, I certainly feel that way, and I do not consider myself unique. Depending on how you view the sport, you can continue to improve as a marathoner forever.

3. TO WIN

To win is the goal of the elite runner, but "winning" (in its narrow definition of "crossing the finish line first") is a goal only a tiny percentage of runners will ever achieve. In my long career, I have won four marathons overall but have won my age group on numerous occasions, including a gold medal in the M45 class at the 1981 World Masters Championships.

My early wins came relatively easily. Decades ago in the United States, the typical road race attracted at best a few dozen participants. If you were a reasonably competent runner, the odds were decent that you might cross the finish line in first place sometime if you trained properly and chose the right race. In some of the smaller marathons, you still may be able to claim a first, or at least achieve an age-group victory if you break 3:00 (for a man) or 3:30 (for a woman).

In today's marathon scene, with race fields as large as forty thousand and first-place cash prizes of $100,000 or more, the odds of crossing the line first have diminished considerably. Usually only the top ten earn prize money. A small number of tightly focused runners might earn an award for finishing high in their age group. Most people return from a completed marathon with no more than a race T-shirt and a medal or certificate that is given to all finishers. They earn their victories when they maximize their potential. And this in itself may be a more significant victory than merely crossing the finish line first.

BASE TRAINING

The first rule for anyone starting his or her first marathon is to set a goal of merely finishing. Select a pace and shoot for a time much slower than you think possible, just to get a finish under your belt. I repeat my frequently stated expo advice: *"Start slow!"* After achieving the "victory" of a finish, then—and only then—should you contemplate training harder to finish faster.

Almost anyone in reasonably good health can finish a marathon. The distance of 26 miles 385 yards is not that far when you think about it. By walking at a comfortable pace of 3 mph, you could cover the distance in about 9 hours. Not many people would be waiting around to greet you, but you could finish. Achilles International in New York helps runners with disabilities to finish marathons with honor. I remain humbled at the achievements of the Achilles runners. More and more people, particularly those in the various charity training programs where the principal goal is raising money rather than finishing fast, choose to walk rather than run.

Recognizing this, at least a few marathons provide early starting times (1 to 2 hours earlier) for walkers and slower runners, including Grand Rapids, Fox Cities, Little Rock, and Maui Oceanfront. But several marathons, including three listed in an earlier edition of this book, have discontinued the practice. This includes Flying Pig (Cincinnati), Bermuda, and Avenue of the Giants (Bayside, California). Early starts are not always popular with faster runners, forced late in the race to pass walkers and slower runners. The faster runners complain, and race directors respond by discontinuing the practice.

You can continue to improve as a marathoner forever.

On one occasion, when I was running a (catch-up) marathon a month so I could run my 100th marathon at the 100th Boston Marathon in 1996, I accepted an early start at Bermuda. A group of several dozen not-as-slow-as-me runners surged ahead, but eventually I caught them and moved into the lead—or into the lead of the early-start runners. It felt good leading a marathon again, although eventually the faster runners from the main field caught and passed us.

Starting early offers mixed blessings. One problem is that there may be few volunteers on the course to assist you before the main race begins. But that still beats being stuck on the course long after everybody has headed home. Toward the end of the Chicago Marathon, policemen in squad cars move relentlessly past the slowest runners, requesting that they move to the sidewalk. Given the necessity in a big city of returning the streets to the citizens, it is a reasonable request to make of those whose splits indicate they will miss the 6:30 official course closing. Chicago warns its entrants: "Those who finish outside of the time limit will not be recorded as official finishers and may not receive full on-course support from aid stations and traffic safety personnel." Some marathons close their courses earlier than 6:30; a few stay open until everyone finishes. If you are worried about finishing within a specific time period in your chosen marathon, check to determine race policy, which usually is stated on the race website.

Do not even think BQ.

Slow runners are accommodated much better today than they were when Kenneth H. Cooper, MD, author of the bestselling book *Aerobics*, ran Boston in 1962. Ken remained out on the course with the clock approaching 4 hours. His wife, Millie, needed to plead with officials to remain long enough so Ken could get an official time. Contrast that with the present day: The last finishers in the Honolulu Marathon, one of the few races in which the officials wait for everybody, usually come in at around 15 hours! That is a slow walking pace.

Realistically, how fast might a runner new to the sport be able to finish a marathon? By jogging as well as walking, you should be able to move at a speed of 4 mph. That pace will get you to the finish line in under 7 hours. Slow running is not necessarily easier than fast running. For one thing, you remain out in the sun longer. Marathon champion Bill Rodgers once said respectfully about those in the back of the pack, "I can't even imagine what it's like to run for 5 or 6 hours."

With a little more conditioning and determination, you can run at a pace of 12 minutes per mile, or 5 mph. At this rate, you could complete the marathon in close to 5 hours, which is a reasonable goal for a "fitness jogger" who wants only to finish.

Moving into the 4-hour or 3-hour bracket requires more training, and getting into the 2-hour bracket requires both training and talent. Nevertheless, impossible goals sometimes prove possible. Most people, of course, never come close to achieving the times of the running elite. As marathons increase in size and more and more people of different abilities realize that lack of speed is no impediment to participation, median times decline. The slowest marathon recorded may have come one year at Honolulu, when one man took more than 29 hours! (He fell, was injured, went to the hospital, and returned the following day to finish.)

Although statisticians find it convenient to talk about median or average times, I like to believe that there are no average runners. I consider us all above average—at least as individuals. When you even begin to consider the possibility of finishing your first marathon, you move well beyond anything that might be described as "average."

The better prepared you are, the better trained you are, the more you'll enjoy your marathon, particularly if it is a first marathon. That's common sense. I don't need a scientific survey to defend the truth of that statement. Runners know this. Even nonrunners about to become runners know this.

But what some runners, even some experienced runners, don't always know is what to do for the weeks and months immediately before committing themselves to one of my 18-week programs.

Here is the training program you've been looking for: Base Training. Looking for a program to develop your base fitness before starting a marathon program? This is it. If you have time before your 18-week program begins, use this 12-week program to get ready so that you will be able to take the 6-mile long run in Week 1 of your marathon program in stride.

Base Training: Novice

Week	Mon	Tue	Wed	Thu	Fri	Sat	Sun
1	Rest	1.5-mile run	3-mile run	1.5-mile run	Rest	30-min walk	3-mile run
2	Rest	1.5-mile run	3-mile run	1.5-mile run	Rest	30-min walk	3.5-mile run
3	Rest	1.5-mile run	3-mile run	1.5-mile run	Rest	30-min walk	3-mile run
4	Rest	2-mile run	3-mile run	1.5-mile run	Rest	30-min walk	4-mile run
5	Rest	2-mile run	3-mile run	2-mile run	Rest	30-min walk	3-mile run
6	Rest	2-mile run	3-mile run	2-mile run	Rest	30-min walk	4.5-mile run
7	Rest	2-mile run	3-mile run	2-mile run	Rest	30-min walk	3-mile run
8	Rest	2.5-mile run	3-mile run	2-mile run	Rest	30-min walk	5-mile run
9	Rest	2.5-mile run	3-mile run	2.5-mile run	Rest	30-min walk	3-mile run
10	Rest	2.5-mile run	3-mile run	2.5-mile run	Rest	30-min walk	5.5-mile run
11	Rest	3-mile run	3-mile run	3-mile run	Rest	30-min walk	3-mile run
12	Rest	3-mile run	3-mile run	3-mile run	Rest	30-min walk	6-mile run

This Base Training Program was designed for novice runners, those new to the sport. For more experienced runners, you will find Intermediate and Advanced Base Training versions on my website.

WHY DO WE RUN MARATHONS?

Committing yourself to a race of 26 miles 385 yards is not a frivolous decision, not merely because of the difficulty of running that far but also because of the time and difficulty of training to run that far. In an Internet poll, I identified some of the more popular reasons nonrunners decide to become runners and marathoners. Respondents were allowed to select multiple reasons they started. Surprisingly, "raising money for charity" failed to be a major motivator.

Had been running shorter distances, moved up	11.5%
For motivation: "If I can do this, I can do anything"	11.5%
Inspired by others who ran marathons	10.3%
To get in shape for health reasons	9.2%
To lose weight	5.8%
To cope with divorce or other lifestyle change	5.8%
In memory of someone	5.8%
Bucket list: something I always wanted to do	4.6%
For mental health	4.6%
To challenge myself	3.5%

5

Ten Marathon Truths

The Simple Facts of Marathon Life

Those who follow me on Twitter often have a unique way of signaling their agreement to comments I often make.

They tweet back, "Truth!"

Truth seems like a good mark to aim for as I interact with runners seeking advice. The marathon is not a complex event. You do not have plays like in football; you do not have signals like in baseball. You line up on point A, and 26 miles 385 yards of running later, you finish at point B. But learning how to maximize performance between those two points often can take dozens of marathons run over a period of years and years.

Truth!

After coaching an uncountable number of marathoners, I feel that just maybe I have learned how to help runners both train for and run the marathon correctly. Here are ten marathon truths that will help you in your next race.

TRUTH NUMBER 1: PROGRESSIVELY LONGER RUNS ENSURE SUCCESS.

Runners using my programs begin 18 weeks before a marathon with a series of weekly long runs. Novice runners start at 6 miles, intermediate runners at 8, advanced runners at 10. The maximum long run is 20 miles 3 weeks before the race, with novices running this distance once, intermediates twice, and advanced runners three times. Scientists sometimes refer to this approach as *progressive overload*. Each week you run a little bit farther than the previous week and train your body to cover what once seemed like incredible distances.

Sounds simple? Actually, it is.

Although the end point for the last long run may be slightly different, most training programs center on similar, progressive buildups. Bill Wenmark, a Minnesota coach, sometimes lets his most experienced runners (those who have run ten marathons) go as far as 30 miles for their longest runs. Jeff Galloway of Atlanta pushes his groups to 26 to 28 miles. On the short side, Jack H. Scaff, Jr., MD, founder of the Honolulu Marathon, considers 15 miles far enough for first-timers—provided their goal is only to finish. When I talk with runners outside the United States, where distances more often are measured in kilometers rather than miles, I sometimes suggest 30 kilometers (18.6 miles) as a more than acceptable maximum training distance because it is a round number. (The training programs on my website have handy, one-click buttons that translate miles to kilometers.)

The purpose of training is to break the body down so it will rebuild itself stronger than before.

Numbers aside, what all programs have in common—other than a loving, hands-on approach—is the graduated progression. The mental benefits of completing a 20-miler at the end of the training period probably equal the physical benefits.

During this months-long buildup for the marathon, weekly mileages increase along with the length of the long runs. Novices in my program more than double their weekly mileage from 15 miles to 40 miles. For more advanced runners already training 40 miles weekly, an increase of 50 percent to near 60 miles is common. Where you end in weekly mileage depends partly on where you begin.

TRUTH NUMBER 2: REST DAYS DO KEEP YOU HEALTHY.

Mileage buildups of the magnitude required to finish a marathon create stress. I'm not going to lie to you. Run 20-milers too often, and even the most experienced marathoners start to hurt. Welcome to the world of stretching and cross-training that we use to heal our injuries, or perhaps more correctly, help us ignore that we injured ourselves by doing too much too soon.

A certain amount of stress is acceptable and good because it creates strength. Too much stress, however, is bad. Many runners condition themselves mentally and physically to run every day, with few days off to rest. This may be all right if you run easy, training for health and enjoyment with an occasional 5K thrown in for spice. If you are peaking for a marathon, however, failure to take rest days is a ticket to injury.

The purpose of training is to break the body down so it will rebuild itself stronger than before. The musculoskeletal system generally requires 48 hours to recover after hard work. It's when you fail to allow time for this rebuilding phase that problems occur. Overtraining can result in muscle injuries and stress fractures that halt training or in upper respiratory illnesses and frequent bouts of fatigue that limit performance. Research suggests that runners at peak training depress their immune systems and thus become easy victims for any germs floating around. In other words, *Ah-choo!* This is particularly true for the weeks immediately before and after a marathon. David C. Nieman, DrPH, a professor of health and exercise at Appalachian State University, did the classic study that proved that runners in the weeks immediately before and immediately after their marathons got more colds than nonrunners.

To avoid the stress that comes with overtraining, bracket the hardest workouts of the week (specifically, the long runs) with easy days and/or days of total rest. Intelligent use of cross-training (walking, swimming, cycling) offers another way to reduce the stress of the marathon buildup.

TRUTH NUMBER 3: TAKE ONE STEP BACK TO TAKE TWO STEPS FORWARD.

Taking rest days is not enough to guard against the dangers of overtraining; most successful marathon programs also include rest weeks in which runners cut mileage, particularly of the weekend long run. The late Chuck Cornett of Orange Park, Florida, promoted a marathon training program in which every fourth or fifth week featured a 50 percent drop in mileage. My programs moderate the long run every third week. Portland's Bob Williams suggests a 25 percent mileage backup every other week, particularly as mileage mounts toward the end of the program: When you get up around 16 miles for your long run (or 40 miles of weekly mileage), some people can't handle that level of stress. It can become a grind. Long runs on the weekend are supposed to be fun. If you begin to dread them, you're working too hard.

Psychological recovery is as important as physiological recovery. Running 20 miles in a workout the first time may be euphoric, but it is also emotionally draining. You can slow down to go the distance, but you are still spending a lot of time on your feet. Merely focusing your mind to place one foot continuously in front of the other for several hours at a time can be exhausting.

Regularly scheduled step-back weeks make it possible to survive the stress load that is part and parcel of the high mileage necessary for successful marathon training. You can relax during step-back weeks, knowing that you are storing strength to push ahead to the next level of achievement.

TRUTH NUMBER 4: SPEED TRAINING CAN BE A DOUBLE-EDGED SWORD.

Elite runners all use speedwork to fine-tune their training. Fast runners—those who finish behind but not too far behind—also understand the benefits of combining intensity with endurance. But most runners are happy just to finish comfortably in a reasonably good time and thus do not need sophisticated training methods. Speed training gets in their way. The extra leg fatigue can make doing the vital long runs much more difficult. It is one stress too many, sometimes even for experienced runners. Elite runners often spend 20 minutes or more a day working on the flexibility required to run fast. Beginners do not have time for that.

Psychological recovery is as important as physiological recovery.

Other forms of exercise can be even riskier. Many first-time marathoners come to the sport of running from complementary sports, such as soccer or volleyball, or they participate in aerobics classes. Strength training can improve your overall fitness, but you do not want to start anything new during your marathon buildup, and some activities need to be eliminated until the marathon is over. Doing a long run in the morning and attending a spinning class (or even a yoga class) in the afternoon is not a good idea. During the taper period immediately before the marathon, you also need to cut back on any supplementary exercises.

TRUTH NUMBER 5: LEARNING TO PACE AND LEARNING TO RACE REMAIN CRITICAL SKILLS.

Almost anybody can run 26 miles if they run at the right pace. Finding that right pace is not as easy as it seems. Run too fast and you'll crash. But run too slow and you may achieve a less than satisfactory performance. Thus, my "run slow" strategy works only if you do not run too slow. Experienced runners eventually must learn to fine-tune their pace to achieve peak performance. The goal for many experienced runners is *negative splits*, running the first half slightly slower than the second half. In other words, someone hoping to finish in 4 hours would go through the first 13.1 miles in 2:00:01 or slower and hope to do the second 13.1 in 1:59:59 or faster. This is not easy because course profile and weather conditions can have an immeasurable effect on your pace. The Boston Marathon is a race with downhills at the start and some pretty tough uphills two-thirds of the way into the race, just when body systems are beginning to crash. If runners get lured into a too-fast early pace, those uphills may prove tougher than need be. You do not want to arrive at the base of the hills exhausted. Running a fast first half might get you to the finish line faster on certain occasions, but that strategy entails some risk, since even a slight miscalculation can result in failure.

Consistency is critical to success in the marathon.

Marathoners often talk about *banking time*, running a faster-than-average pace in the first half of the race so that if you start to slow in the second half, you can still reach your goal pace. In my mind, this is a very risky strategy.

The pacing teams that have become popular in many marathons take a lot of the guesswork out of staying on pace. One way to fine-tune your pace is to include some training at race pace during your buildup. Whether your pace is 6:00 miles (2:37 at the finish) or 12:00 miles (5:15 finish), you need to know how it feels to achieve that pace. My intermediate and advanced training programs include pace runs on Saturdays before the long runs on Sundays.

Most novice runners, however, do not know their marathon pace because they have never tested it in a marathon and many have not run races at shorter distances. Running occasional races will help you test your limits and determine your approximate marathon pace.

TRUTH NUMBER 6: CONSISTENCY RULES THE DAY.

Extra-long runs, including those 30-mile long runs mentioned earlier, do not always work. Or at least they do not work if you have not nudged your mileage up over a period of months and even years so such pinnacle workouts can be handled without excessive strain. In all training matters, consistency counts. Consistency with a purpose is critical to success in the marathon. The gradual buildup of a lot of miles turns a 5K runner into a marathoner. In my novice program, Tuesdays and Thursdays are easy days, when runners go only 3 to 5 miles, most often running at a conversational pace.

This sounds like a "throwaway" workout, one you could eliminate from your schedule without damaging your fitness much. But you cannot. Every workout is important. Consistency in running each workout is most important. Even running 3 miles at an easy pace, you are burning close to 300 calories, checking out your system, loosening your legs to ready yourself for the next hard day's training. From messages posted online, I know that many runners take pride in following my training schedules precisely as they are written, day after day, week after week, month after month. If they miss even a single day, they wonder if they have compromised their training. Have a wedding scheduled one weekend? They ask my permission to do the long run the weekend before or the weekend after. One runner from Salt Lake City once wondered if he could do his Saturday long runs on Mondays, when he had the day off. Sure, I said. And it is okay to flip-flop workouts and weeks, just as long as you do not lose too many pieces from the puzzle.

Is this anal behavior? I guess so, but consistency in training always worked for me, and it should work for you, too.

TRUTH NUMBER 7: GOOD NUTRITION MAKES GOOD RUNNERS.

Yes, everybody knows that runners are supposed to eat pasta the night before the marathon to maximize glycogen storage, but if you pay attention to what you eat only for that one meal, you never will succeed as a runner. You need to eat correctly before your long runs in training, too—and every single day of the week! Eating intelligently is one more key to marathon success. If you make poor food choices, you compromise your ability to train hard—or even to train easy. You also miss the opportunity to train your intestinal tract to manage food and fluids while running. Consistency works in training, and consistency works in nutrition, too.

That does not mean you cannot have an occasional burger with chips and wash it all down with a mug of beer, but the most successful marathoners follow diets that contain around 55 percent carbohydrates, 30 percent fats, and 15 percent protein. That ratio works for good health, too. Forget what you read about low-carb diets. Low-carb diets may offer some short-term weight-loss benefits, but they simply do not work for endurance athletes.

That does not mean spaghetti seven nights a week. Other good sources of carbohydrates, according to sports dietitian Nancy Clark, RD, author of *Nancy Clark's Sports Nutrition Guidebook*, are cereals, fruits, juices, breads, rice, plain baked potatoes, peas, corn, fruit, yogurt, and frozen yogurt.

But not ice cream, cheesy lasagna, and pepperoni pizza. No, no, no! Those foods often get confused with carbohydrates, but they actually contribute more fat than needed to your diet. "Carbo-loading should begin months before the race, not the night before," advises Clark.

TRUTH NUMBER 8: PRACTICE ALL THINGS CONNECTED WITH THE MARATHON.

The purpose of the long runs is not merely to get your legs in shape but also to get the systems around those legs in shape. A critical item for running success is learning to drink on the run and finding the proper combination of water and replacement drink that works best for you. And if your marathon of choice has a specific replacement drink, you'd better practice drinking that, too. You do not want to get to the first aid station only to discover you do not like the taste of what's provided. There is no exact formula for how much or what to drink, since that depends not only on individual runners' preferences but also on weather conditions. On very warm days, you probably will choose more water than sports drink.

Make your mistakes in workouts or unimportant races.

You definitely also need to learn what foods may upset your stomach if eaten the night before or the morning of a race, and avoid them. That is another reason that some racing is necessary during the marathon buildup. You need to get used to the race experience: how to warm up, where to pin your number, what it feels like to run in a crowd, whether your shoes will cause blisters. Make your mistakes in workouts or unimportant races, so that you can make corrections for marathon day.

Once you decide on your race day strategy, stick with it. Do not make sudden changes. An old cliché states: "You gotta dance with the one that brung you!"

TRUTH NUMBER 9: TAPERING IS BOTH AN ART AND A SCIENCE.

Not every coach agrees on how many days or weeks before a race to begin resting. And maybe we should not agree, the runners we coach being individuals. Depending on the person—and the race distance—the pre-race taper can vary from 3 days to 3 weeks. I recommend a 3-week taper, although when I was running my fastest times and logging 100 miles a week, I tapered 10 days before the marathon, with the final 5 days featuring little or no running.

Tapering not only permits the healing of any damaged or fatigued muscles but also promotes maximum glycogen storage. You do not want to go into the race with your leg muscles even slightly depleted of glycogen.

Although mileage drops during the taper, the speed at which you run that mileage should not. The taper period is a good time to practice race pace but at much shortened distances. One way to cut mileage is to convert easy days into days of complete rest. You may want to jog easily the day before the marathon just to reduce nervousness, but do not go too far. Arrive at the starting line rested and ready to go.

TRUTH NUMBER 10: MINUS MOTIVATION, YOU WILL NEVER SUCCEED.

Listen up, everybody: Motivation needs to come from within. People sometimes underestimate the effort it requires to run 26 miles 385 yards. Finishing a marathon requires courage and commitment. If running marathons were easy, everybody would be doing it. You need to be committed to your training. If you are not focused on being a success, you will not be successful. You will never succeed if you are not willing to prepare. End of lecture.

If you find it hard to motivate yourself, enlist others to help encourage you. This could include friends and family whom you keep posted on your progress. Start writing a blog. Even if nobody reads the blog, your commitment to put words on paper (or hurl them into cyberspace) can help carry you through those tough days in August when the miles get long and the weather gets hot. Or enroll in a class. One of the greatest class benefits is runners supporting each other.

Running 26 miles 385 yards is one activity for which it is true: You get back what you paid for. Runners willing to train properly, taking careful note of the ten truths listed in this chapter, will find that the marathon can be an experience that provides much more joy than pain.

WHAT THEY LEARNED WHILE TRAINING

When I asked runners participating in social media what lessons they learned while training for a marathon, I got these responses.

Kenny Baldo of Manalapan, New Jersey, learned that he was not Superman and if he did not listen to his body, he would break down: "Running could be my kryptonite, or it could be my salvation."

Martin Van Walsum of Carlisle, Massachusetts, learned that the success of a training plan was highly dependent on the sum of its parts: "Every run has its purpose."

Doug Spence of Houston, Texas, learned that once you find a formula that works, do not change until it fails you: "That includes food, clothing, sleep, and good-luck charm."

Amber Balbier of Dallas, Texas, learned to swallow her pride and stop running workouts as if they were races: "I need to keep the easy runs easy, so the hard runs can be hard."

(continued)

Martin Schumacher of Chicago learned patience: "I can't force my training. I just have to let it happen and come to me."

Dave Stubbe of Chicago learned that training is a series of peaks and valleys: "Don't get too excited about the peaks or too down about the valleys."

Wendy Miller of Bloomington, Indiana, learned that scheduled rest days are just as important as regular workout days: "Adding a mile here and a mile there gets you into trouble."

Tom Hughes of Fremont, California, learned that undertrained is better than overtrained: "Run slow in training, stick to the mileage, and don't be afraid to cut a run short or take an extra rest day if the body demands it."

Kathy Olney of Acton, Massachusetts, learned that no single workout is crucial: "The cumulative effect of many workouts makes the difference."

Kristine Nader of Chicago learned about herself: "I can do more than I ever thought I could."

Nick Morris of Madison, Wisconsin, learned that no matter how well your training goes, things can happen on race day that prevent you from attaining your goals: "Take what you learned, and move on to the next training cycle."

6

Striving to Improve

Becoming a Better Runner

How do you improve as a marathoner? How do you run faster? These are key questions for many runners. Getting to the finish line of your first marathon is just a matter of preparation. Either through talent or with the help of a well-structured and progressive training program (or both), most people who set their minds on becoming marathoners succeed. It's all about motivation.

If these new runners become hooked on the sport, their next goal is to get better at it. They seek to run their fastest marathon, whether it is their third or their thirty-third race. It is not that simple, but it is also not that difficult.

If you are a beginning runner who has just finished your first marathon, you will continue to improve if you do nothing else but train consistently. Most established training programs for first-time marathoners last 3 months or more. Class leaders guide their students through a graduated schedule, the main feature being a long run that gets progressively longer (usually moving upward from 6 miles to 20 miles) as marathon day approaches. Students are then sent to the starting line undertrained and well rested because experience has shown that to be the best way to ensure that they finish.

It works!

Better to be safe than sorry. And who can argue with success? Thus, most well-coached first-time marathoners run their races without the training necessary to achieve peak performance. They run comfortably slower than their talents might allow. Remember my previously reported expo exhortation: *"Start slow!"* First-timers finish the race thinking they probably could have run somewhat faster if they had trained harder. They are right. They can. And so can you.

Even without adopting a refined training schedule, most marathoners can improve merely by continuing to train at or near the same level. After 3 months, you will have only begun to reap the benefits of that level of dedication. Your undertrained body will continue to improve, as long as you do not overtrain it.

Here's the key. Keep doing some running in the middle of the week. An hour is a good length for at least one midweek workout. Run somewhat longer on the weekends: 90 to 120 minutes, although no more than two or three times a month. Take 1 or 2 rest days weekly, as suggested in my novice training schedules. Fill in the rest of the week with runs at various short distances, and mix in some running at near your marathon pace. The accumulation of miles over a period of time will help you improve. You will get better. That's a promise!

1. CONSISTENCY

Consistency is a word you already have encountered several times in this book, and I am not through using it. I cannot emphasize enough the importance of maintaining consistency in your training. Consistency does not mean running 20-milers every weekend; it does mean maintaining a base level of fitness even when you are not training for a specific race.

Research by Edward F. Coyle, PhD, of the department of kinesiology at the University of Texas at Austin, suggests that runners begin to "detrain" (lose their fitness) after 48 to 72 hours and that it takes 2 days of retraining to regain the fitness lost for every single day of training that is skipped. That does not mean you should never rest, but if you take extended periods off, it will take you longer to come back.

Not every runner wants to hear that. When I have quoted Coyle's research online from time to time either on my Facebook page or in a tweet, I sometimes get brushback from individuals who object to hearing that the 18 weeks of hard work done preparing for a marathon may be gone forever if they don't continue training at least at a somewhat lower level.

You will get better. That's a promise!

I need to remind them that consistency is critical to marathon success. You do not need to maintain continuous peak condition, but settle on a consistent level of training that you know you can maintain for 12 months of the year. When it comes time to aim for a specific marathon or half marathon, you can increase your level of training—slightly. The important thing is to maintain an effective endurance base.

The ACSM guidelines for fitness suggest 3 or 4 days of exercise a week, 20 to 60 minutes a day. That's the minimum fitness formula for maintaining good health, beyond which Kenneth H. Cooper, MD, president and founder of the Cooper Institute in Dallas, Texas, suggests you are exercising for other reasons. For the marathoner, that will be true: Your reason is to stay in shape to run marathons. You will need—and want—to run more than the time allotted in Dr. Cooper's formula. But the basic pattern offered in the ACSM guidelines still applies to marathoners.

For four years, I coached the boys' and girls' cross-country teams at Elston High School in Michigan City, Indiana, and I also worked with the distance runners during the track season. Between seasons, many of us ran together as much for fun as for fitness. I encouraged my runners to keep diaries, and I tried to examine the entries periodically to monitor the students' conditioning programs. I discovered that the less dedicated ones would train hard for 3 or 4 days, but then they would miss 3 or 4 days of running. They thought they were staying in shape, but they were actually sliding backward—as they proved when they appeared for practice the first day of the season. The students who trained consistently improved; the others did not.

As a result, I told them this: Never go 2 days without running. One day of missed training is no problem. That qualifies as rest. But 2 or 3 lost days in a row (taking into account Dr. Coyle's research) equals lost conditioning—and inevitably will mean poorer performances once the season begins.

2. FINDING YOUR MILEAGE LEVEL

At peak training, most elite runners average 100 miles or more a week. You cannot compete successfully as an elite runner in the marathon, or even as a near elite, unless you run a lot of miles. During my best years, that was my mileage goal for just before my most important races, but maintaining that level is not easy. Most runners would crash if they attempted to run 100 miles weekly or even half that many miles. Determining the level that is best for you is tricky and may take several years of experimentation, but once you have reached a comfortable level, you can reap the benefits of success.

The best way to determine your optimal mileage level is to keep a training diary, as I advised the Elston runners. Most runners now use computer diaries that allow you to record everything from your mile splits to your heart rate to a map of the course you ran. (I even have an app that provides daily workout data while I offer encouraging words: "One mile to go. You can do it!") Or you can simply mark mileage on a wall calendar.

Never underestimate the power of a simple calendar sheet attached by magnets to your refrigerator. The advantage of even a simple diary is that when things go wrong—or right—you can analyze your training and determine the reasons. Those older, upstairs training diaries, recording several decades of workouts, fill a full shelf of the bookcase in my office and prove very valuable when I am writing articles for *Runner's World* and books such as this.

During special periods, such as when I was preparing for a marathon or peaking for maximum performance at the World Masters Championships, I would take poster board and a black marker and make my own diary calendars showing 3, 6, or 9 months—whatever the training for that particular race required. I would tack the poster-size calendar to a cork wall in my basement that I passed each day before and after running. It served as both a visual record of what I had done and a reminder of what I had to do. In addition to what I wrote in my diary, I would mark weekly mileage totals and sometimes specific key workouts, such as the distance of my long run.

I used my record-keeping system as motivation but also as a safety net. If I noticed that I had run 4 consecutive weeks at too high a mileage level, that would trigger a reaction: *Hmm. Maybe I should back off my training for a week to avoid getting injured.*

Finding the appropriate training level is not easy—particularly because that level may change as you get stronger or older—but it is essential if you want to improve as a marathoner.

3. SLOWING IT DOWN

If there is one difference between fast runners and those who finish at the back of the pack, it is that the fast runners seem to have no qualms about running slowly. They are not embarrassed about it. One year at the Boston Marathon when I was in town appearing at the expo but not running the race, I went out the day before for an easy jog of a few miles along the Charles River. Returning, I arrived at a pedestrian bridge across Storrow Drive at the precise moment two Kenyan runners arrived.

I had seen them at a press conference the day before, so I smiled and nodded, and they smiled back. After we crossed the bridge and continued to jog up a side street toward our hotels, I realized I was jogging faster than they were! In fact, I had to slow my pace to avoid embarrassing myself by passing them. The following day I saw them on TV at the front of the lead pack. If runners capable of sub-2:10 marathons are not embarrassed to jog very slowly, you should not be, either.

Finding the appropriate training level is not easy.

The important message is not that fast runners often run slowly but that they train *differently* each day. If I had to cite one mistake made by inexperienced marathoners when they seek to improve their performance, it is that they run too many of their miles at the same pace and over the same distance. There is little variety, and that limits their improvement.

If I am running slowly on one day, it is probably because I ran hard the day before—or want to run hard the next day. To improve, you need to add intensity to your program. You may not necessarily need to run sprints on the track, but you need to run at least as fast as race pace. Very few runners can run race pace day after day. In order to train at a high level of intensity on certain days, most of us need to train at a low level of intensity on other days. That's where slow running comes in.

From a scientific standpoint, slow running is important for two major reasons.

Caloric burn. This varies from runner to runner and depends on size and metabolism, but many of us burn 100 calories for every mile we run. Burn 3,600 calories by running 36 miles and you lose 1 pound. It almost doesn't matter how fast you run those miles. You can even walk and burn a large number of calories per mile. And if your form is awful compared with that of smooth-striding elite runners, the more calories per mile you probably burn. Scientists quibble over the precise numbers, but calorie loss is related to foot-pounds: the amount of effort (that is, energy) it takes to push a body of a specific weight forward. One means of attaining maximum performance is to achieve optimal body weight and an optimal percentage of body fat. You can do that just as easily with long, steady distance: It will take you somewhat longer than if you ran those miles fast, but you will be less likely to become injured.

Sparing glycogen. Exercise physiologists say that when you run slowly, your body has time to metabolize fat as a source of energy. When you run fast, your body burns glycogen, a derivative of carbohydrate, as its preferred energy source. Glycogen is stored in the muscles and is a more efficient fuel, in the sense that the body can metabolize it more rapidly than fat. (That's one reason why we marathoners favor a high-carbohydrate diet.) But by training slowly, you apparently teach your muscles to become more efficient at also metabolizing fat, thus sparing glycogen stores for those last few miles in the marathon.

4. REST IS BEST

Certainly, those three words sound cliché, but I keep using them online while answering questions from runners wondering whether to run or rest the next day if fatigued or injured. "Rest is best." I figure that if you need to ask whether to take a day off, you probably already know the answer and are only waiting for me to confirm your choice: "Yes, rest is best."

Not running is as important a part of the marathoner's training guide as resting. That may sound somewhat confusing at first, but running a short distance at a slow pace would qualify as "rest." A day when you cross-trained by swimming or cycling also might qualify as rest. My rest day when I was averaging 100 miles a week was 8 miles up and down the Lake Michigan beach in front of my home in the morning and 8 miles again later that afternoon. And, yes, those runs were resting compared to what I did on my hard days. But sometimes active rest is not enough; you need to take a day off when you do not run or do much of anything. Although I promote consistency as critical to success, there are times when you simply have to kick back and do nothing. And I mean nothing! You need to be consistent about resting as well as training. Take a week off. Take a couple of weeks off. Yes, you will lose some fitness, but you will more than make up for it when you return to training refreshed and ready to run hard again.

Following my victory in the marathon at the World Masters Championships in New Zealand one year, I flew home with no future goals. I took 2 months off. Two full months off! This was after a year and a half of intense training, when I frequently did those 100-mile weeks. It was not so much that my body needed that period of extended rest; my mind needed the rest. Okay, I did a lot of cross-country skiing during those 2 months, but that isn't cheating too much, is it?

Knowing when to back off and take off a complete day—or even more—is one of the secrets of marathon success. It is not easy, since the traditional work ethic that has proved successful for many people suggests that more is better. That training calendar on my basement wall would be more of a hindrance than a help if it pushed me to run extra miles just to achieve mileage levels I might have planned months ago—without considering whether I have a cold, failed to get enough sleep the night before, or am overly fatigued because I spent most of the previous day on an airplane.

Sometimes you need to take a day off.

Rest is essential to success. In my training schedules, I program 2 days of rest into each week for first-time marathoners. Most experienced runners understand that tapering before a marathon—cutting training mileage the last week or two before the race—is important to ensuring success. Less recognized is the necessity for rest and mini tapers all through the marathon training program. Take a day off; it won't hurt.

Does this message contradict the earlier one related to consistency, the importance of maintaining a steady schedule? Not at all, because who can better afford to take days off than someone who trains consistently?

If you hope to get better as a marathon runner, you need to pay attention to the basic elements—consistency, mileage, intensity, and rest—but those are only four of the routes available to you. Let us consider next the benefits and challenges of building up mileage.

7

Building Mileage

How Many More Miles?

The experts agree: Building up weekly mileage is essential for achieving success in any long-distance event, particularly the marathon or half marathon. You need time on your legs. You need to develop pace awareness. You need to learn how to control your mind as well as your body. You need to figure out how to manage nutritional needs. You need to condition yourself to remain vertical while moving relentlessly forward for long periods of time: 3 or 4 or 5 or 6 or more hours, the runner's equivalent of *To infinity and beyond!* But how many weekly miles are necessary in order to achieve this level of conditioning?

In a survey of coaches conducted for the first edition of this book, the general consensus was that 35 miles a week was adequate if your goal was only to finish a marathon, 55 miles to finish well. Most elite runners believe 100-mile-plus weeks are necessary to excel, but some research suggests anything more than 75 miles a week may be a waste. That much mileage most certainly is a waste for 99 percent of those running marathons today.

A second survey of runners who followed me online showed that 42 percent thought they had run too few miles before their most recent marathons, and 58 percent thought they had hit it right. Nobody felt they had run too much!

How many miles do you need to run each week? It depends on your goals, your abilities, and your schedule—and, in some cases, on whose advice you're taking.

Before the 1980 U.S. Olympic marathon trials in Eugene, Oregon, a survey of the American contenders showed that nearly all of them trained more than 100 miles a week—somewhat disheartening for the aspiring marathoner now doing 15 miles a week and hoping to work up to 50 or more.

> **It is less how many miles you run than what you do with those miles.**

Bill Rodgers and Frank Shorter, 1976 Olympians and two of the most successful and consistent American road racers of their time, trained 140 miles a week. "I always felt best when doing high mileage," says Rodgers. Alberto Salazar ran 130 miles a week before the 1984 marathon trials. Portugal's Carlos Lopes, the 1984 Olympic champion, ran 140, on average. Joan Benoit Samuelson, the women's gold medalist in the 1984 Games, also ran more than 100. Norway's Ingrid Kristiansen ran as many as 125 miles weekly prior to breaking Samuelson's world record in the 1985 London Marathon.

But not every elite distance runner thinks you need to run so many miles. Don Kardong of Spokane, Washington, finished fourth in the 1976 Olympic marathon (2:11:16) with less mileage than most top marathoners, averaging 80 to 90 miles most weeks. "My feeling is that people pick 100 because it's a nice, round number," he says. "But 88 is an even rounder number."

Consider Benji Durden, a top runner from Boulder, Colorado, and a coach of elite and midpack runners. When he ran 110 miles a week at an average pace of 6:30 per mile, Durden had PRs of 29:21 for the

10K and 2:10:41 for the marathon, and he made the 1980 U.S. Olympic marathon team.

But Durden found the stress of that much training too intense. In 1983, he cut his mileage to a still-demanding 85 to 95 miles a week—and set new PRs. He improved to 28:37 for the 10K and 2:09:58 for the marathon, finishing third at Boston. "I believe you can be a successful performer on low mileage, as little as 70 to 80 miles a week," Durden now says. Granted, most of us would not consider 70 to 80 miles a week low mileage, but it is for an elite runner.

Yet by the end of the millennium, American distance runners—once dominant on the world scene in the era of Shorter, Rodgers, Salazar, and Samuelson—had become second-rate performers. Kenyans, who sometimes run three workouts a day, fill the front ranks of most major marathons. In 1997 and again in 1998, the New Balance shoe company put $1 million on the line for any American man or woman who could break the national record. Although the U.S. women's record of 2:21:21 set by Samuelson was then very close to the world record, the men's mark of 2:08:47, set by Bob Kempainen, was "soft," nearly 2 minutes off the world record. Nobody collected the prize. The closest anybody came was Jerry Lawson, a high-mileage runner, who ran 2:09:17 at Chicago in 1997. Then Lawson failed to complete three of his next four marathons.

More recently, Americans have begun to return to the podium (top three finishers) at major international races, if not always occupying the top step. Meb Keflezighi and Deena Drossin Kastor won silver and bronze medals, respectively, in the marathon at the 2004 Olympic Games in Athens. Galen Rupp placed third in the marathon at the 2016 Olympics in Rio de Janeiro. Shalane Flanagan won the 2017 New York City Marathon. Amy Cragg placed third in the marathon at the 2017 IAAF World Championships in London.

Meb and Deena (as they more often are called) proved that it is less how many miles you run than what you do with those miles. In the 9-month buildup to the Olympics, the pair averaged 120 to 140 miles a week, high by any standard, but Deena emphasized that it was not the quantity of miles but the quality that resulted in their strong showings. "Over a period of years, I had matured as a runner," Deena says. "This permitted me to increase the intensity of my training. That's what took me to the next level."

MAINTAIN YOUR BASE

Although most recreational runners cannot even comprehend the talent and training required to reach weekly mileage levels of 120 to 140, let's skip the first digit. You can make significant improvements if you maintain your base at 20 to 40 miles a week. Train comfortably at that level over a period of time, solidify your ability to do long runs between 10 and 20 miles, and then you can concentrate on intensity to improve your bests at all distances. What's interesting about Deena's training is that during the winter, she ran many of those miles using snowshoes.

Both Deena and Meb did much of their training at Mammoth Lakes, California, where the altitude of 8,000 feet made it difficult to run fast. Deena often would drive down the mountain in the morning for workouts several thousand feet lower, below the snow line. Afternoons, she often would don snowshoes and go to 9,000 feet for runs through the woods. "If you live in a ski area, you need to learn to embrace winter," she says. "The mechanics of running on snowshoes are slightly different, but there's less impact, plus stopping in a snowy meadow beneath a fir tree and taking in the mountain scenery is a great way to relax the mind and avoid the tedium of all that high-mileage training."

Do runners whose goals fall somewhat short of an Olympic medal need to run lots of miles? If your goal is merely to finish with a smile on your face, do you need to punish yourself by running long not only on the weekends but also during the week to push your mileage up into the stratosphere? The answer is both yes and no.

Scientists agree that high mileage helps you better use glycogen, the starchlike substance stored in the liver and muscles that changes into a simple sugar as the body needs it. Carbohydrates in the diet are our main source of glycogen—one reason spaghetti is such a popular prerace meal for marathoners. Glycogen is the preferred fuel for running, but your levels can become depleted within 60 to 90 minutes. Thereafter, your source of fuel becomes fat, which is metabolized less efficiently.

Many ultramarathoners (those who race at distances beyond 26.2 miles) believe that a "keto" (high-fat) diet can help you teach your body to burn fat more efficiently. As a proponent of high-carbohydrate eating, I strongly disagree.

Succeeding as a high-mileage runner takes more than diet.

Nevertheless, high-mileage running teaches your body to burn more fat along with the glycogen, stretching your reserves from 60 to 90 minutes up to 2 hours or more. Top marathoners such as Meb and Deena are efficient in metabolizing both fats and glycogen throughout the length of their races (because of the vast volume of their training) so that they rarely deplete their stores. As a result, they do not hit the wall.

Succeeding as a high-mileage runner takes more than diet, however. William J. Fink, a researcher at Ball State University's Human Performance Laboratory in Muncie, Indiana, suggests that volume training may result in a more efficient use of muscle fibers. "When a runner doubles his training mileage, we often see no change in his maximum oxygen uptake, the ability to deliver oxygen to the muscles," explains Fink. This, he says, indicates that something else—perhaps improved muscle fibers—causes the better performances.

Jack H. Wilmore, PhD, the late exercise physiologist and professor emeritus in the department of kinesiology and health education at the University of Texas at Austin, suggested there is a psychological effect to high mileage as well. "When you do 100 miles a week, your legs are chronically fatigued," he once told me. "Then when you finally do taper before an important race, it makes you feel all the stronger. The same would hold true for a 30-mile-a-week runner who, through a gradual buildup, achieved an ability to train comfortably at 60."

Dr. Wilmore claimed that all those miles help your body adapt to the punishment that occurs during marathons—in ways that scientists cannot yet explain. "When I'm out of shape and I race at long distances, everything hurts," he said. "It feels like my connective tissues are coming apart. But when I'm ready for a marathon and have put in the miles, everything moves smoothly."

So what does all this mean to those of us who dream of qualifying for Boston or setting a new PR? "There's no mystery about how you improve your endurance," says Lee Fidler, a running coach from Stone Mountain, Georgia, with a marathon PR of 2:15:03. "You just increase volume. I ran 110 miles a week 10 years in a row, but not everybody can do that. For most people, 60 is plenty."

But for someone running his or her first marathon whose weekly mileage may (gulp) have been expressed in single digits before sending in an entry blank, the thought of running 60 miles in a single week may seem frightening, while 110 weekly miles ranks as beyond comprehension. The average reader of *Runner's World*, according to surveys by that magazine, runs 20 to 25 miles a week. When preparing for a marathon, that same individual bumps that mileage by another 10 weekly miles. My Novice 1 marathon training program peaks at 40 miles in its climactic Week 15, but runners reach that lofty goal in only that one week. In the half-dozen weeks before the peak, the weekly mileage is in the 30s.

WEEKLY MILES

Most of us who call ourselves runners, who pride ourselves on our dedication to the road-running sport, run more than a few weekly miles. In a survey I conducted of my online followers, I found that 15 to 25 miles a week was the most popular distance.

(continued)

How Many Miles Do Marathoners Run?	Percentage
15 miles a week or more	23%
16 to 25 miles a week	37%
26 to 50 miles a week	32%
51 miles a week or more	8%

Although you can finish a marathon on only 30 miles a week, in order to finish well, you may need to push your mileage up to near the 60 miles that Fidler suggests. My intermediate training programs peak near 50 weekly miles; my advanced programs, closer to 60. From feedback, I know that some veteran runners feel my mileage levels are low, that they might achieve more if they pushed up to 70 or 80 or 90 or more weekly miles. "Fine," I tell them, "but I absolve myself of all responsibility if you train too hard and crash."

Still, I concede that the marathon veterans have a point. There comes a time when you need to wave goodbye to the coach who got you started and plunge forward on your own. Brian Piper, founder of the Chicago Marathon training class, was running 70 miles a week when he broke 3 hours and qualified for Boston.

When Brian and I worked together to develop the training programs used in that class, we concentrated on keeping the mileage buildup gradual: no more than a mile a week for the long runs, 2 miles a week for the weekly mileage. Every third week, we had runners under our charge step backward (cutting a few miles off the long runs) to recover. If you increase mileage constantly week after week, you get stronger, but you also risk hitting your breaking point. Brian and I felt it best to approach that point without reaching it. We taught runners in the Chicago class to go up two steps, drop back one step, then jump up two steps higher, a seesaw route to marathon success.

A brief warning: Counting calories does not always work if you hope to lose weight, and counting miles does not always work if you hope to score a marathon PR. What you need to beware of is concentrating on how many miles you're running to the exclusion of everything else. Some runners become fixated on high mileage, feeling that if they fail to reach their weekly mileage goals, they remain unfulfilled. They begin worrying by Wednesday or Thursday: "Am I going to make it this week?" At this point, they're running more for their training diaries than for themselves. They are also spending a lot of time running "junk miles"—miles that have no effect on fitness or performance.

Although high mileage may help produce better times, simply adding mileage may not guarantee success for either the world-class athlete or the dedicated fitness runner who dreams of one day running the Boston Marathon. Quality must be mixed with quantity to produce maximum results. This is the risk that comes with keeping a running diary: You become very concerned with how many miles you ran this week but not with how fast you ran them. The late David Martin, PhD, a U.S. Olympic team consultant from Atlanta, believed that much of the so-called rehabilitative running that elite

> **Quality must be mixed with quantity to produce maximum results.**

runners do between hard runs may simply deaden their legs. "One of the secrets to remaining fresh," he says, "is to limit impact time, the number of times your feet strike the pavement."

Some runners jump from 50 to 75 miles to the "magic" 100 simply by adding a second workout to their day. Dr. Martin had his doubts about the gains from multiple workouts, particularly for near-elite runners. "Run 5 miles each morning, multiply that by 7, and you get 35 miles," he said. "If you add that to 65 miles of hard training in the afternoon, you can write 100 in your training diary. But does that make you a better runner?"

Dr. Martin continued: "It is not how much training you do as much as it is how well you recover from it. Because if you do not recover adequately, you will become either injured or sick or chronically fatigued, with resulting poor performance. Thus, while everyone has a different number of miles per week that they can tolerate (due to weather, terrain, biomechanics, lifestyle) without breakdown, the secret to success is not to exceed that threshold."

Invariably, people who achieve the highest level of success for their ability—regardless of whether they are winning marathons or merely running in the middle of the pack—are those who minimize the destructive effects of high mileage and maximize the efficiency of the miles they run.

THE RED LINE

Top marathoners talk about *redlining*, a term borrowed from auto racers. The redline is the mark on the tachometer that delineates the safety zone from the danger zone. If you consistently rev your engine higher, it disintegrates. If you are a NASCAR driver, you need great results because that new engine is going to cost your team up to $110,000.

In running, redlining means pushing your training to achieve maximum efficiency and your best performances. But if you push past your redline regularly, you risk injury or breakdown. The cost of a visit to an orthopedist or podiatrist to fix that injury fails to match the NASCAR engine replacement cost, but you want to avoid any injury that can be prevented.

A beginning runner might redline after a gradual buildup to 30 weekly miles. Or 45. Or 60. There are physiological limits: I hate to scare you, particularly if you are a newbie, but running too many miles too soon results in injuries, such as strained tendons and ligaments, stress fractures, chronically tired legs, and a persistent feeling of fatigue.

There are also psychological limits. Some runners cannot cope with dressing, running, and showering all the time—as well as the need for extra rest. Not only does 100 miles weekly require 10 or more hours of actual running time, it also requires a lot of recuperative time. Elite runners probably need 3 to 4 hours of rest daily on top of 7 to 8 hours of sleep each night. That's fine if you are a professional runner with promises of a six-figure paycheck if you win one of the major marathons, but most of us are amateurs for whom running is a hobby.

Scientists have not been able to define the precise point—between undertraining and overtraining—where optimal benefits occur. And this point certainly differs among athletes. One runner may thrive on 30 miles a week, another may need 60, and a third may need 120 to excel. The optimal mileage level may also change at different points in a runner's career. I consider this especially true when it comes to masters runners. Past age 40—and particularly past age 60—you simply cannot train as hard or as much as you could as a youngster.

In general, runners who can increase training mileage should expect to improve as long as they do not sacrifice quality for quantity. The key is to increase mileage gradually and pay careful attention—very careful attention—to how your body reacts.

8

Running Long

The Most Important Workout
You Will Do

The long run is the staple of every distance runner's diet. It is the single most important workout you do each week. If you are a seasoned marathoner, workouts up to 20 miles are de rigueur. If you call the homes of most distance runners on a Saturday or Sunday at 7:00 a.m., you will find they are either already out running or just about to head out the door. Running long will get you ready to perform.

In my programs, first-time marathoners use a single 20-miler as a confidence builder before tackling the full 26 miles 385 yards. Intermediate and advanced runners do multiple long runs as one means of improving their PRs. Even 5K runners find that regularly running long helps them run faster. And if you are interested only in fitness, a longer-than-usual training run with friends on the weekend can be fun.

But what is the purpose, in both physical and psychological terms, of the long run? What function does it serve in getting you ready for a half or full marathon? What is the perfect distance for running long, how often should you do it, and at what pace should you run?

Most experienced runners and their coaches agree that running long is not only enjoyable but also essential to achieving success in distances from 5K to the marathon. "The single long run is as important as high mileage in a marathoner's training program," says Alfred F. Morris, PhD, from Washington, D.C. Tom Grogan, a coach from Cincinnati, ranks it second only to "raw talent."

Coach Robert Wallace of Dallas, a 2:13 marathoner who placed ninth at Boston in 1982, says, "I still love those long, easy runs on Sunday. They're the mainstay of any training program. You don't get results immediately. It's like saving pennies: Put them in a jar, and over a year you accumulate $50 to $60."

Wallace favors slow workouts rather than fast ones for the long runs. "High-quality [fast] runs are too hard on a weekly basis," he says. "Run low-quality and you can get out every weekend. I like to see 10K runners go 14 to 16 miles; marathoners go 20 to 22 miles, several minutes slower than race pace."

Running long offers a dress rehearsal for the race.

Joe Friel of Scottsdale, Arizona, who coaches runners in person and online, considers the long run essential for building an endurance base. Friel has his runners do at least one long run every week or every other week. "Every 10 days would be perfect," he says, "but that's tough to fit into a work schedule."

David Cowein, an ultramarathoner from Morrilton, Arkansas, runs long once a month for 2 to 6 hours. "I'll usually run trails," he says. "If I did a run that long on roads, I'd be sore the next day, but trails are easier on my body. I'll run far, but I'll also run slowly, walking up hills if necessary."

Runners often do their long runs in groups. "It's great to run with a group because it can be lonely out there," says Wallace. "Even when I ran fast times, I always trained with slower runners. I just wanted to run long and didn't care at what pace."

While working on an article for *Runner's World* many, many years ago I posed some questions on long runs to a number of top coaches. Each coach agreed that the long run was the key to marathon success. "Shun long runs in training and you'll pay the price for your neglect," warned Al Lawrence of Houston, a former world-class runner from Australia (bronze medalist in the 5,000-meter race at the 1956 Olympics). But not all coaches surveyed agreed on every detail of marathon preparation. Here is what the top coaches had to say about running long.

1. WHY DO WE DO LONG RUNS?

Running long offers a dress rehearsal for the race. "It's a test," says John Graham, who coaches runners on the Internet.

Florida-based coach Roy Benson agrees: "Running long gets you used to the stress of lifting your feet up and down nearly 5,000 times per hour. It allows you to practice skills you will need in the race, such as taking fluids. Long runs build confidence in your ability to succeed, and, maybe equally important, you learn patience."

"Many runners push too hard on daily runs," says Bob Glover, who supervised coaches for New York Road Runners. "The long run forces them to slow down and pace themselves wisely—just as they must do in the marathon."

But apart from practical and psychological considerations, there are strong physiological reasons to run long. Robert H. Vaughan, PhD, an exercise physiologist who trains both elite athletes and first-timers for the BMW Dallas Marathon, offers some important advice:

> The long run serves to increase the number of mitochondria, as well as capillaries in the active muscles, thereby improving those muscles' ability to remove and utilize available oxygen. In addition, the long run recruits muscle fibers that would otherwise go unused. This recruitment ensures a greater pool of conditioned

fibers that may be called upon during the later stages of the race. There are certain psychological barriers and adjustments to central nervous system fatigue that also are affected by the long run.

That advice is deep and difficult for a layperson to understand—but it is also the single most important reason you should run long.

2. HOW LONG SHOULD YOUR LONGEST LONG RUN BE?

When in gathering information for this book I asked this question on Twitter, the answers came ratcheting back: "20." "20." "20." I thought I was in an echo chamber, but then again my Twitter followers more often were using my marathon training plans with a maximum distance of 20 miles for the long run. Nichole Swiger of Nashville, Tennessee, courageously said 22 miles for her first marathon, but 18- to 20-mile long runs for marathons after.

There is no "perfect" distance. Twenty miles is the peak distance used in most training programs, if only because 20 is a round number. That is the peak distance I suggest in all my training programs—even for advanced runners. But in countries outside the United States, 30 kilometers (18.6 miles) is equally round and as frequently used. Most coaches feel that once you reach 16 miles, you are in long-run territory, and I agree. Twenty is the point where the psychological and physiological changes mentioned by Dr. Vaughan kick in. But a few coaches prefer prescribing "time" rather than distance: hours rather than miles. Coach Benji Durden points to 3 hours as the equivalent of running 20 miles.

That was probably true in the 1980s and into the 1990s, when the median time for most marathoners was around 4 hours. Today, with increasing numbers of marathoners taking longer than 4 hours to finish, stopping short may not be enough. For a first-timer hoping to finish in 6 hours, a 3-hour workout would result in only about 13 miles of running, hardly enough to condition that person for the full distance. Common sense must dictate whether you choose time or distance to measure your long runs.

A more-than-common-sense approach might be to sometimes use 20 miles as the end point for your long runs and sometimes use 3 hours. If running off the road, such as on the mountain trails above Boulder, Colorado, where Benji lives, time versus distance makes most sense to me.

Running much longer increases the risk of injury, particularly for first-timers. For experienced runners, the suggested top number is about 23 miles, according to coaches to whom I addressed the maximum-distance question. And that distance actually was my long distance for many years, but only because a nearby course was 23.2 miles long.

Coach Glover peaks first-timers at 20 miles and experienced runners at 23 miles—but also puts a cap at 4 hours of running, regardless of how many miles you've covered. "The goal," says Glover, "is at least three long runs of 18 to 20 miles for novices and five or six runs of 20 to 23 miles for experienced runners."

Coach Jeff Galloway peaks participants in his nationwide training programs at 26 miles—but they do a lot of walking to get that far. At the far end of the spectrum, elite Japanese runners do 5-hour runs, which probably take them past 30 miles. Former world record holder Rob De Castella and his training partner Steve Moneghetti, both Australians, used to peak with a 30-miler 5 weeks before the marathon, but that was after a steady diet of 23-milers nearly every weekend. Most runners would self-destruct on that much mileage. At one point in my career as an elite athlete, I pushed the distance of my longest runs up past 30 miles, seeking increased endurance, but I failed to reap any benefits. Runs that long simply took too much time and increased my fatigue level.

Coaches feel once you reach 16 miles, you are in long-run territory.

The greatest danger, however, is that doing long runs much longer than 20 miles increases the risk of injury. I have no studies or hard data to prove this point, but based on my prior experience I strongly believe it to be true. I continue to be haunted by the memory of a party I attended one year before the Chicago Marathon. One woman hoping to run Chicago as her first marathon had followed a program designed by another coach that peaked at 26 miles. In her last long run a month before the race, she pulled a muscle at 24 miles and had to stop. "What a shame," I thought. If the same had happened in the actual marathon (which the injury forced her to miss), the woman surely would have been motivated enough to walk or limp the final 2 miles and earn her finishing medal.

Nevertheless, I do not disagree with Coach Bill Wenmark of the Twin Cities, who encourages his most experienced runners to push past marathon distance for their longest runs. Wenmark defines "experienced" as having previously run ten or more marathons, someone who probably regularly runs 50 to 60 miles a week. If such a marathon vet experiences an injury and loses training time—or maybe even misses the race—it is not as shattering an experience as it would be for someone doing their first marathon.

What was that advice I offered a few chapters ago? *"Start slow!"*

3. HOW OFTEN SHOULD YOU DO LONG RUNS?

Mike Korfhage of Louisville, Kentucky, suggests three long runs, spaced out a few weeks apart in any training cycle. That's true, and even my Novice 1 program prescribes a 16-mile run in Week 11; an 18-mile run in Week 13; and a 20-mile run (finally) in the climactic Week 15. I consider runs 16 miles and above to be true "long runs," but let's concentrate on 20-milers.

If you are a novice following my program, you run only one long run at peak distance: the traditional 20-miler mentioned previously. Nearly every training program gradually builds runners up to near that distance, rests them for 2 to 4 weeks, and then sends them off to the starting line. And it works! Most runners who follow the marathon training schedules on my website jump fairly easily from 20 miles in practice to 26 in the race. The excitement of the event coupled with several weeks' rest during the taper period helps them bridge the gap. First-timers often surprise themselves when they discover that running the marathon can be almost easier than training for it. (That is assuming you train for it correctly.)

But finishing that first marathon and racing subsequent marathons are two different beasts. To improve, you probably need more long runs, not merely longer runs. Experienced runners do not need to emulate the Aussies mentioned earlier and run 23-milers every weekend, but in the closing stages of their preparation, they probably need to run between three and six workouts that are between 18 and 22 miles, according to the marathon coaches I consulted.

As with novice marathoners, the reason is psychological as much as physical. "The more peak-distance runs runners achieve in their marathon preparation, the more confidence they radiate," states Bob Williams, who prepares runners for the Portland Marathon.

Run long too often, however, and you raise your risk of not only injury but also staleness. Only experienced runners should venture often into that 18- to 22-mile window, and even they risk making mistakes.

4. WALKING BREAKS: YES OR NO?

Here's where I encountered some disagreement. Not all the responding coaches bought the idea expressed in an April 1998 *Runner's World* article by Amby Burfoot titled "The Run/Walk Plan." Burfoot recommended that taking regular walking breaks is helpful both in workouts and in races.

"No!" thundered one coach.

"I thought the name of the magazine was *Runner's World*, not Walker's World," grumbled another.

Al Lawrence was the most diplomatic dissident. He said, "Runners seem to feel better about themselves when they say 'I've *run* a marathon,' rather than 'I've *done* a marathon.'"

That was the reaction in 1998, but as we moved into the new millennium, most coaches began to concede that walking is not that bad a strategy, particularly if your goals are less than Olympian. When you are running 10:00 miles or slower, the difference between that pace and a brisk walking pace may not be that much.

And just because you break to walk in a marathon, that does not mean you are a slow runner. A brief walking break (notice that I said "brief") may actually allow you to gather yourself and continue at a faster pace. On a warm day, I ran a 2:29:27 and won an M45 title at the World Masters Championships, walking through each aid station. My son Kevin used the same strategy to run 2:18:50 and qualify for the 1984 Olympic trials. Bill Rodgers walked several times and even stopped to retie a shoe while winning the 1975 Boston Marathon in 2:09:55. So no apologies needed, you walking runners.

> **Doing long runs much longer than 20 miles increases the risk of injury.**

Kristen Farrell of New Jersey tells me that she is more likely to take a break to hydrate or stretch or just as a breather than to actually walk in a training run. "I take breaks mainly so as not to overdo it during training runs," she says.

I also need to nod to my colleague Jeff Galloway for his success in promoting walking breaks for his runners. Some of Jeff's followers walk a minute for every 10 minutes run. Others, whom I have encountered in marathons, run 30 seconds and walk 30, an approach that would have been called "scout's pace" when I was a Boy Scout.

On one occasion, a magazine journalist approached me for an interview for an article she was writing on "Higdon vs. Galloway," about the difference in our approaches in training marathoners. But I consider Jeff a friend and feel that we are maybe 98 percent in agreement when it comes time to coaching runners, especially first-time marathoners. Jeff pushes his runners a few miles farther than I do mine, but he trains them for longer periods than I do.

Also, rather than tightly prescribing "Run Walk Run" breaks, I suggest to my runners that they walk through aid stations. With aid stations a mile apart in many marathons, the result is about the same.

COACHES TELL ALL

Runners differ in their backgrounds and abilities. There is no single workout or training program that works best for everyone—and this certainly is true when it comes to doing long runs. Yet in surveying coaches, I did find a consensus about how far and how often a person should run long, specifically during the marathon buildup. The numbers differ according to whether you are a first-time marathoner or an experienced runner hoping to better your time at that distance. Here is what the coaches advise.

Category	First-Timers	Experienced
Longest run	20 miles	23 miles
Frequency	1 time	3 to 6 times
Pace (per mile)	Race pace	30 to 90 seconds slower
Weekly mileage (max)	40 miles	55 to 60 miles
Walking breaks	Okay	Maybe
Speedwork	Nope	Definitely yes

To summarize the feeling of the coaches on two important issues: Walking breaks are okay in a marathon if your main interest is in finishing and you do not care about time. Experienced runners seeking to run fast, however, may want to skip the walk breaks (except through aid stations to ensure proper fluid intake). Speedwork (training faster than race pace) is considered too risky for first-timers. Experienced runners who do their long runs slower than race pace are likely to benefit from midweek speed sessions, including long repeats at race pace.

If you do plan to walk during long runs or in the marathon itself, here is how and when to do it.

- It is a good idea to walk through aid stations. You can grab more fluids and drink more easily while walking.
- Walk if you cannot run any farther, although it's best to walk before you're forced to.
- Do some walking in training, if only to learn how to start running again after being brought to a halt.
- Take walking breaks in training and races if the coach of your program tells you to do so.

5. HOW MUCH RECOVERY AFTER RUNNING LONG?

Ntutu Letseka states: "Personally I recover quicker from long runs than other quality efforts." He suggests that within 36 to 48 hours he is good to go again.

Dr. Vaughan, meanwhile, summarizes the consensus of the coaches I interviewed when he says, "An experienced marathoner with years of training may recover in 48 to 72 hours, while a novice may require 2 weeks." Most runners in training will benefit from a day's rest after doing their weekend long runs, and probably an easy day after that, before taking another hard workout at a shorter distance. Thus, we arrive at the following pattern.

Sunday: long run
Monday: rest or easy run

Tuesday: easy run
Wednesday: hard run

That does not mean that the "hard" run on Wednesday should be another 20-miler. Most first-timers should probably choose a medium-length run of between five and ten miles for their midweek (hard) workout. In coaching marathoners, I describe this as the "sorta-long" run (a term I borrowed from Olympic marathoner Julie Isphording). Experienced runners may be more likely to do their next fast (hard) workout on either Tuesday or Wednesday.

> **"Drinking during workouts is as important as drinking during races."**

Most marathon training programs, including mine, allow 2 weeks between long runs near peak distance. The programs schedule medium-long runs (10 to 14 miles) on the weekends between.

Rest before the long run is as important as rest after. If you program a day or two of easy running and/or rest before your long runs so that you are not overly fatigued prior to them, recovery afterward will be easier. This is particularly true for first-timers.

6. AFTER THE RUN, ANY TRICKS TO RECOVERY?

Annie Burke of Boynton Beach, Florida, boosts the regenerative properties of a nap. An hour's nap will do, says Burke. "It totally regenerates my mind and body."

Other than that, there are no tricks, just sound training and nutritional practices. The three best strategies cited by our coaches were gels, energy bars, and massage. Use the first two during the long runs, the last after. "Taking gels and bars during the long runs speeds recovery," says running guru Joe Henderson, author of two dozen books, including *Marathon*

Training. "You need to keep your glycogen stores continuously high if you want to maintain training effectiveness."

Bob Williams considers dehydration to be one of the major sources of muscle soreness and also a source of muscle cramps during long runs. "Drinking during workouts is as important as drinking during races," he says.

Massages can be expensive, but when you decide to train for a marathon, you make a major time commitment and also a financial commitment, considering the cost of entry fees, not to mention the cost of travel if you pick a marathon not in your hometown. Given that commitment, you might as well do right by everything connected with the marathon. Schedule a massage for 48 hours after your long run, since that's often the peak point of muscle soreness. The massage will help you ease your way back into your regular routine. More frequent massages during the final 6 weeks leading up to your peak long run may help reduce the risk of injury by keeping you loose and relaxed. For that reason, massages also work well as preventive therapy 24 hours before a hard workout or long run. (A nod to Julie Sosa in Indiana and Lori Nicholas in Florida, my regular massage therapists.) Typically, I schedule a massage every other week. In the closing stages of marathon preparation—or if any problems develop—I may get more frequent massages.

7. HOW FAST TO RUN DURING LONG RUNS?

This is an important question and an equally important answer. Speed is of limited importance during long runs. More important is time spent on your feet. One long-run strategy for runners following time-based programs is to set as their goal for the longest run approximately the length of time they plan to run in the marathon itself, not worrying about the distance or the speed at which they cover the distance. That is handy if you plan to run on unmeasured courses, particularly ones that would take you off roads and into the woods. "Sub-2:10 marathoners [who race faster than 5:00 pace] have been known to run their long runs at over 7:00 per mile," says Dr. Vaughan.

Novices in most training programs connected with major marathons run the same pace in their long runs as they will run in the race. "That's because we encourage first-timers to select a conservative time goal to guarantee their finish," says Bill Fitzgerald, one of the leaders of the Chicago Marathon training class. He adds, "If you can't hold a conversation during the closing miles of your long run, the pace probably was too fast."

Maybe how fast you run on a week-to-week basis is not that critical. Matt Williams of the London-based Serpentine Running Club nails it when he says, "Run slow enough to chat with your running companions, or slow enough to enjoy being outdoors." Bob Glover says the same more rhythmically: "If you can chatter, the pace doesn't matter."

Experienced marathoners who continually run long at race pace can get into trouble unless they slow down. They risk both injury and overtraining. Although the law of specificity suggests that you need to do some running at race pace to condition your muscles to the specific pace you will attempt to hold in the marathon, this is best accomplished during midweek workouts at shorter distances. "It's better to err on the slow side," Al Lawrence suggested.

On several occasions, I've experimented by doing long runs at race pace or faster, wondering whether it might make me stronger. I found that I could maintain this level of effort until the long runs got up to about 12 or 13 miles. After that, I began to encounter problems, the most serious being an inability to maintain the quality of my workouts during the rest of the week because of failing to recover fast enough. It became an example of robbing Peter to pay Paul. With Paul looking at the cash handed to him and saying, "You owe me a few quid more."

But consider this fact: Not every long run needs to be done at the same pace, nor does the pace within each run need to be the same. Coach Denis Calabrese believes runners should do the second half of their runs faster than the first half, both in practice and in the actual marathon. "The discipline of going out slow rather than allowing the excitement of the marathon to burn you up is very valuable," says Calabrese.

Didn't I say, *"Start slow"*?

For experienced marathoners, I often recommend the 3/1 approach taught to me by New Zealand's John Davies, bronze medalist in the 1500 meters at the 1964 Olympics and a respected disciple of Coach Arthur Lydiard, also from New Zealand. Davies advised doing the first three-quarters of a long run at a slow pace, then picking up that pace in the last quarter—although not quite to marathon pace. In a 20-mile run, this would mean slow for the first 15 miles and faster for the final 5 miles. Davies did not recommend converting every long run into a 3/1 effort. He felt once every second or third week was sufficient.

How slow is slow, and how fast is fast? If you are looking for numbers, do your long runs 30 to 90 seconds per mile (or more) slower than the pace per mile you expect to run in the marathon. Notice that I qualified the time prescription with "or more," meaning I really do not care how slow you run, as long as you cover the distance—and there are exceptions even to that. Always be aware that inclement weather can render irrelevant any plans to train at a specific pace over a planned distance. Fatigue from activities related to your life away from running also can be a factor.

Not every long run needs to be done at the same pace.

In a 3/1 workout, you might run the first three-quarters at a pace 90 seconds or more slower than marathon pace, then pick up to 30 seconds slower. But that is getting almost too precise for comfort. The most important point is to run slow enough at the beginning of a long run so that you can run somewhat faster at the end. This strategy works well in the actual marathon, too.

8. CAN 5K RUNNERS BENEFIT FROM LONG RUNS?

Dave Weber of Glen Allen, Virginia, says: "Not sure what the science shows, but my best 10Ks have come post-marathon training."

The scientists say to keep training like a middle-distance runner. In fact, all the coaches I surveyed agree. "Endurance is a factor at all racing distances," says Joe Henderson. "Even 5K and 10K runners can benefit from 1- to 2-hour runs, but anything much longer might drain energy away from their more specific speedwork."

Running long regularly also is an effective way to both lose a few pounds and maintain weight. Do not overlook the psychological value of a regular, weekly long run, particularly if it gives you an opportunity to run in the company of friends whom you might not get a chance to see during the week. One reason that many runners continue to sign up for marathons is that preparing for that long distance provides both focus and structure to their training. It gives them an excuse to do long runs, which is something they want to do anyway. Whatever the reason, the long run is here to stay as a regular part of our training regimen.

WHY RUN LONG?

The weekend long run remains the most important workout in our quiver of training arrows. But different runners have different reasons for running long, as I discovered when I surveyed those who follow me on Twitter.

Emily Graves, Corinna, Ontario: You run long to take you near 42.2 kilometers, but leave you hanging in suspense at the 32K mark. It's progressive physical, physiological, and mental conditioning.

Michael Wix, Auckland, New Zealand: To help the body adapt to sustained periods of exertion similar to those of your race.

Twila Johnson, Gresham, Oregon: To have more time to reflect on why you love running and what it does for your spirit. That time allows you to observe the beauty of the world around you rather than just the path you're on.

Andrew Wilson, Los Angeles, California: The long run is a race simulator. It's key in helping your body and mind adapt to being out there for hours on end. As someone who loves running for hours, it's a run to look forward to every weekend.

Ryan Koenig, Pittsburgh, Pennsylvania: If you are a runner, the long run is what you look forward to all week. It can be incredibly difficult, but when you finish you know you've done something. And then next week, somehow, you'll go even farther.

Meredith Caballero, Wichita Falls, Texas: They make my shorter runs seem so easy.

Ajay Thombre, Dubai: Long runs train the body and mind to stay on their legs for a longer period of time. Nutrition can be planned and practiced for race day. The same applies to the running gear. Breakfast and coffee taste better post run.

9

The Half

13.1 Miles en Route to 26.2

The half marathon, the "half," 13.1 miles, 21.1 kilometers, remains an important distance even for those who run and race twice as far. Many individuals come into the sport and choose the half as their first race distance, en route to the marathon, or for others 13.1 miles may be the longest distance they ever run. In most of my marathon training programs, I suggest running a half marathon in Week 8 or Week 9 (out of 18 weeks), as a checkpoint, a place to pause and get your bearings and also determine what you might expect for a finishing time when you reach the end of your 18-week program.

A poll by Running USA suggests that 44 percent of runners consider the half marathon their favorite race. This is borne out by registration numbers collected by that organization: 508,000 runners registered for marathons in 2018, with four times that number (2,090,000) registering for half marathons.

This does not mean that runners have begun to abandon the full marathon. Participation numbers for both distances have remained about the same for the last half-dozen years. Twenty-six point two remains the Holy

Grail, the highest-status running magnet to attach to the rear of your car. But we successfully integrate half marathons into our racing schedules. This is particularly true among women; 57 percent of the finishers in half marathons are female, compared with 41 percent of the finishers in marathons. And it is not because women are "weak" and cannot go the full 26.2. "They just like the distance," says Jason Jacobson of Running USA.

But there are other reasons for the explosion of interest in half marathons. Here are the three groups most likely to choose 13.1 miles as a road-racing option.

1. NEW RUNNERS NOT YET READY FOR PRIME TIME

Committing to a 26.2-mile race with its 18-week buildup is a significant step, particularly if you are new to the sport and maybe just a little bit out of shape and overweight. Getting into shape and losing that weight is one reason people decide to start running. They will achieve more success if they select an achievable goal, but does that goal need to be 26.2 miles of racing? Not lately, and newcomers have many more racing options, the most popular currently being 13.1 miles. The half is a goal that a newcomer can see on the horizon rather than over the horizon. Yes, I know: The term in large print on the cover of this book is *marathon*, not *half marathon*, but the half offers an easy-entry test to determine whether that newcomer has the mojo for a full marathon.

I applaud this approach—and, in fact, have been suggesting it for years. As I viewed the new generation of runners, it always seemed far from ideal that the marathon was often the first race they would run. To me, that was like skipping high school and going straight to college, missing some of the fun along the way. (No prom?) As diplomatically as pos-

> **"Deciding to run my first half marathon changed my life."**

sible, I would suggest to these so-called newbies asking questions about marathon running: "Before starting my 18-week program, why not run a 5K or a 10K to get a feel for the sport?"

Astrid Haakonstad of Belleville, Michigan, took that route: "My first race was a 5K, then I set my sights on the 10K. Then the half marathon." Only after that buildup did Haakonstad consider the full. She now combines running marathons with shorter races.

Heather Richards of Corinna, Maine, says, "My goal following bypass surgery was the Walt Disney World Half Marathon. I made that goal a reality."

Deborah Margraff of Arlington, Virginia, started running for fitness. "Then I gravitated toward the half and full marathon when I found out it was easier (for me) to go farther than faster."

Alli Mincher of Rochester, New York, adds: "Deciding to run my first half marathon changed my life."

FIRST RUNNING GOAL

"What was the Big Event that attracted you to enter the sport of long distance running? What was your first, immediate goal?" When I asked that question on Twitter, I assumed that most people would automatically respond, "The marathon." I was wrong. New runners began with shorter distance races such as the 5K or 10K and only then lifted their gaze upward to the marathon, the half marathon being an important stopping point along the way.

First Running Goal	
No particular distance	14%
5K or 10K	39%
Half marathon	28%
Marathon	19%

So if you are new to the marathon sport, consider making the half marathon one of your first running races. You will learn a lot about the race and about yourself. Most important, you can determine whether you want to continue moving upward in distance, which brings us to the second group of runners attracted to the half marathon.

2. RUNNERS EN ROUTE TO THE MARATHON, FIRST OR OTHERWISE

Some runners select 13.1 as their maximum distance and go no farther. *'Nuff said* seems to be their motto. On to the next item on their bucket list. But others use the 13.1 distance as a stepping-stone to 26.2. To me, either approach seems reasonable, but integrating a half into the training program for a full has become more common lately. To understand why, consider my popular 18-week training program. Novice runners reach 13 miles for their long run in the eighth week of the program. This offers them an interesting option: If you plan to run 13, you might as well tack on an extra tenth of a mile and do a half marathon race. Doing so will allow you to taste at least some of the thrill that you will experience 10 weeks later in your actual marathon, plus you get a chance to test all systems, including nutrition before the race and fluid management during it. Also, are those shoes you just purchased at the running store going to carry you twice the distance without blisters?

More important is that by racing (not merely running) a half marathon, you can get a good fix on what you might be capable of running in a full marathon. One rule of thumb suggests doubling your half marathon time and adding 10 minutes to get an estimate of your marathon time. Thus, a runner who took 2 hours to run a half would double that to 4 hours and add 10 minutes for an estimated time of 4:10.

Guesstimating worked for runners who, two decades ago, purchased the first edition of this book. In 1993, the 10K was the most popular sub-marathon racing distance. Multiplying your 10K time by a formulaic 4.66

allowed you to guesstimate your marathon capability. Multiplying that time by 5 provided a more conservative if not more accurate estimate.

Inspiration will carry you to the finish line.

Still, using a 10K to predict a marathon time works less successfully than using a half marathon. Today's runners are more computer-savvy than those in 1993, and, rather than guess, they prefer to use one of the many prediction calculators available on the Internet. One I often recommend is the calculator provided by Coach Greg McMillan on his website, mcmillanrunning.com. For example, Greg suggests that a 2-hour half-marathoner could run a full marathon in 4:13:05.

Warning: Both methods—guesstimating and calculating—may result in an unrealistic goal for newcomers. Better to be safe than sorry, so I might advise that 2-hour half-marathoner to not set the bar too high. A time goal of 4:30 for a first marathon would result in a friendlier finish and allow you a chance to set more respectable PRs in future marathons, assuming you decide to stay at that distance rather than moving back down to the half. And a lot of people do just that, bringing us to our final category: runners who favor the half marathon distance.

3. VETERAN MARATHONERS SEEKING SHORTER DISTANCE EXPERIENCES

Veteran marathoners already know they can use a recent half finishing time in combination with previous marathon times to judge more accurately their ability and know what to expect in their next full-distance race. A larger number downsize to the half as a good between-marathons option.

You can wear yourself down if you try to run more than one or two marathons a year. My marathon training programs consume 18 weeks of a runner's attention, and my recovery program adds another 5 weeks, for a total of 23 weeks. Two of those a year equal 46 weeks, allowing little time for training and racing at other distances.

In contrast, my half marathon training programs last 12 weeks, and recovery time can be measured in days rather than weeks. A runner focusing entirely on running half marathons easily could fit a half-dozen races of that length into a year's time without risking overtraining. Marathoners also comfortably can fit halves into their training programs. Just 2 or 3 easy days of taper (instead of 2 or 3 weeks), run your race, then after 2 or 3 easy days of recovery, you're back on the road again and aiming at your main goal, the marathon.

TRAINING FOR THE HALF

Regardless of which of the three categories you fit into, you will find that half marathon training programs mimic full marathon training programs. The main difference is that the numbers are less, both for workouts and preparation time.

On page 318, you'll find my novice training program for the half marathon. The schedule assumes you can run 3 miles three or four times a week. If that seems difficult, consider a shorter distance for your first race—or take more time to develop an endurance base.

Follow the example of Andrea Bond from Charleston, West Virginia, who did not even have a goal when she started to run. "I was just pleased to discover I loved running," says Bond. "And I was curious to see what my body was capable of. A year later I ran my first half, and the following year I ran my first marathon and first ultra, a 40-mile trail race."

The terms used in the training schedule are somewhat obvious, but let me explain what I mean anyway.

Pace: Do not worry about how fast you run your regular workouts. Run at a comfortable pace. If you are training with a friend, the two of you should be able to hold a conversation. If you cannot do that, you probably are running too fast. (For those wearing heart rate monitors, your target zone should be between 65 and 75 percent of your maximum pulse rate.)

Distance: The training schedule dictates workouts at distances ranging from 3 to 10 miles. Do not worry about running precisely those distances, but you should come close. Pick a course through your neighborhood or in some scenic area where you think you might enjoy running. Then measure the course either by car or by bicycle. In deciding where to train, talk to other runners. They probably can point you to some accurately measured courses for your workouts.

Rest: Rest is as important a part of your training as the scheduled runs. You will be able to run the long runs on the weekend better—and limit your risk of injury—if you rest before and rest after.

Long run: The key to getting ready to finish a half marathon is the long run, progressively increasing in distance each weekend. Over a period of 12 weeks, your longest run will increase from 3 to 10 miles. Don't worry about making the final jump from 10 miles in practice to 13.1 miles in the race. Inspiration will carry you to the finish line, particularly if you taper the final week. The following schedule suggests doing your long runs on Saturdays, but you can do them on Sundays or any other convenient day.

Cross-train: On the schedule, this is identified simply as "cross." What form of cross-training works best? It could be swimming, cycling, walking, cross-country skiing, snowshoeing, or even some combination that could include strength training. What cross-training you select depends on your personal preference.

Walking: Walking is an excellent exercise that many runners overlook in their training. I do not specify walking breaks, but feel free to walk during your running workouts anytime you feel tired or need to shift gears.

Stretch and strength: Mondays and Thursdays are the days on which you might spend extra time stretching—and doing some strength training, too. Runners generally benefit if they combine light weights with a high number of repetitions, rather than pumping very heavy iron. If you never have strength trained before starting this program, you might want to wait until you finish your first half.

Racing: It is not obligatory, but you might want to run a 5K and/or a 10K race to see how you're doing—and also to experience a road race if you have not run one before. You will be able to use your times to predict your finishing time in the half marathon, as well as what pace to run that race. I have suggested a 5K at the end of Week 6 and a 10K at the end of Week 9. Local race schedules may force you to modify the program.

Running 13.1 miles is not easy. If it were easy, there would be little challenge to an event such as the half marathon. Whether you plan your half as a singular accomplishment or as a stepping-stone to the even more challenging full marathon, crossing the finish line will give you a feeling of great accomplishment. Good luck with your training.

10

The Full

Moving Up to the Ultimate Distance

Bill Fitzgerald remembers his attitude about people he saw running in the park in the years before he became a runner: "I thought, 'Why would anyone waste their time doing that? It can't be fun.' I didn't see any smiles on their faces."

Fitzgerald was 36. "That's an age when males frequently encounter their own mortality," he comments. Though he had played some sports growing up in suburban Oak Park, Illinois—football, basketball, softball, hockey—Fitzgerald was never quite good enough to make a team. He lived a somewhat sedentary life as a security administrator for Chicago's Water Reclamation District. He had begun to gain weight. "I decided, let's try this thing called jogging," he says.

Fitzgerald went to Portage Park, near his apartment, and started to jog. A sidewalk wound through the park, covering a distance of about a mile. He planned to go one lap—but failed. "I got mad at myself," he recalls. "I vowed to finish that lap. I returned each day and ran just a little bit farther. Seeing my improvement gave me a sense of accomplishment."

When Fitzgerald finally finished a 1-mile lap, he felt like he had "won the Boston Marathon."

Fitzgerald continued to run and eventually completed a 5K race. Friends suggested he run the Shamrock Shuffle, a popular 8K held each spring in Chicago. Uncertain how to train for this longer event, Fitzgerald unwisely doubled his training mileage, got shin splints (a general term for soreness in the front lower leg), and had to miss the race. By the spring of 1989, he had met an experienced runner named C. C. Becker at a local health club. With Becker serving as his mentor, Fitzgerald finished the Shuffle in March as well as a half marathon in April. At that point, he figured he was ready to attempt a full marathon. Becker suggested that Fitzgerald join the Lincoln Park Pacers. The club met Saturday mornings in Lincoln Park. The Pacers would run 5 to 10 miles, then adjourn to a nearby café for breakfast.

"Some guy's starting a class next week."

After one workout, a female runner told Fitzgerald, "Some guy's starting a class next week to prepare people for the Chicago Marathon." Fitzgerald and the woman attended the first meeting of the class in July. About thirty-five runners appeared. The meeting was at O'Sullivan's Public House, "a real Irish shot-and-a-beer joint," recalls Fitzgerald. That "some guy" turned out to be Brian Piper, a computer systems analyst who loved running and hoped to share his love with others. Piper outlined a 15-week training program that included a gradual mileage buildup approaching the marathon. The class also featured a series of clinics with speakers offering nutritional and medical advice. Chicago Marathon race director Carey Pinkowski appeared one week to encourage class members.

Piper, like Fitzgerald, was typical of the new breed of runner attracted to the sport for its fitness benefits. Piper had swum competitively in high school and as a freshman at the University of Iowa. But he quit college swimming because it was too time-consuming and instead began to do some running with members of the track team who lived in his dormitory. "I had to struggle to keep up," he says, "but it established running as an alternative activity for staying in shape."

Nevertheless, a year out of college and working for the Regional Transportation Authority in Chicago, Piper found himself 25 pounds overweight. His motivation was the same as Fitzgerald's: to lose weight and get fit. Piper selected the Chicago Marathon as his goal, then made all the common beginner's mistakes while training and in the race: "I didn't do enough long runs. I ran everything at the same pace. I failed to take enough water. I wore cotton shorts, which resulted in bad chafing. Everything was strictly trial and error. Other than what you read in *Runner's World*, I had a hard time getting good training advice." Piper finished his first marathon in 3:54, but he was forced to walk a lot. "There were a lot of 7:00 miles in the beginning and a lot of 10:00 miles near the end," he admits.

Undeterred, Piper set as his next goal qualifying for the Boston Marathon. It took five years, but in 1986 he finally ran a 2:58:25 at the Twin Cities Marathon and was Boston-bound. He was then 32 years old. "I began to think that there ought to be some way to help first-time marathoners avoid all the mistakes I had made," he says.

Piper suggested that the local running club he belonged to sponsor a marathon training class. That brought Piper and Fitzgerald together at O'Sullivan's: one the teacher, one the pupil. It would be an encounter from which many runners—both in Chicago and elsewhere—would benefit greatly.

STEP-BACK WEEKS

Piper taught runners using a 15-week training program borrowed from the St. Louis Track Club, which offered training schedules for runners whose base weekly mileage was 30 (novice), 40 (intermediate), or 50 (advanced). The program followed a hard/easy approach, featuring 2 or 3 hard days a week and 2 or 3 hard weeks a month. Runners did long runs on Tuesdays, Thursdays, and Sundays. The Sunday runs were the longest. Wednesdays and Saturdays, they ran easy. Mondays and Fridays were rest days. The pattern went as follows:

Monday: No running most weeks for novice runners. Intermediate and advanced runners ran 4 to 5 miles.

Tuesday: Long runs between 6 and 10 miles, with the peak coming in the tenth and twelfth weeks. Intermediate and advanced runners ran somewhat more mileage.

Wednesday: An easy run of 4 to 5 miles for novices. Intermediate and advanced runners did a mile or two more.

Thursday: The second-longest run of the week. The novice buildup went from 7 to 12 miles. Intermediate and advanced runners did more runs at peak distances of 12 and 13 miles.

Friday: No running for novice and intermediate runners. Advanced runners ran 6 miles.

Saturday: An easy run of 4 to 5 miles for each category of runners.

Sunday: The weekend long run, what might be considered the *key* to any marathon training program. Novices began at 9 miles and reached 21 in the twelfth week. Intermediates went from 11 to 22 miles, with three runs over 20 miles. Advanced runners went from 13 to 23 miles, with five runs over 20 miles.

The unique feature of the St. Louis program, and what caught my attention when I later reviewed Brian's training approach with him, was St. Louis's "step-up, step-back" approach to the mileage buildup. Miles did not increase in a continuous ascending line (9, 10, 11, 12, and so forth) but rather in a series of waves: Step up to one level, then step back for recovery, then up to a higher level.

This was the schedule that Fitzgerald and the other thirty-four members of the Chicago Marathon training class followed the first year. In many respects, the approach was similar to what Fitzgerald had done instinctively when he had first started to jog in Portage Park. He had gone a little bit farther each day and grown stronger day by day until finally he could finish a mile. In the Chicago class, he went farther every week until finally he could finish a marathon. All marathon training programs are built on similar progressions.

Fitzgerald finished his first marathon in 3:54—coincidentally, the same time that his mentor, Piper, had achieved in his first marathon eight years earlier. "I finished feeling a lot better than Brian," boasts Fitzgerald. "I had better coaching."

Fitzgerald would eventually qualify for Boston by running 3:20:54. By that time, the training class had expanded to several hundred runners annually. Fitzgerald began to share leadership duties with Piper, becoming co-director. Eventually, the class would grow to three thousand members, training in different areas in and around the city. Drive through Chicago's Lincoln Park on a weekend morning during the summer months and you will see runners swarming like bees on the jogging paths. Many if not most of them are training for the marathon.

> **All marathon training programs are built on similar progressions.**

A major reason for the popularity of the class was its social aspect: runners meeting runners. "It's easier to run in a group, and it's a lot more fun," says Piper. Although running in the 1970s and 1980s may have been the province of baby boomers seeking to delay aging, running in the 1990s became the province of Generation X, whose plan was never to grow old.

And as the class continued into a new millennium, another subtle shift in demographics occurred. Increasing numbers of female runners, daughters of the baby boomers, began to embrace the marathon. "We've got the best dating service in town," hints Fitzgerald. "Where would you rather meet your future spouse: Friday night in some smoky bar or Saturday morning on the jogging path?"

And although enrollees may have begun the class still staying out late on Friday nights, after several weeks they realized that if they expected to run well early the next morning, they would need to head home long before their carriage turned into a pumpkin. Usually this message would sink in by the fourth and fifth weeks, at which point the weekend long runs reach 9 and 10 miles.

Although the step-up, step-back pattern remains the same, the Chicago mileage buildup now differs from that of the original St. Louis program. It has been a gradual evolution, not a sudden change. After the Chicago class's first marathon in 1989, Piper invited me to speak at its awards banquet. Several years later, with the number of participants in both the Chicago Marathon and the class increasing, I became a training consultant for both.

THE MONDAY NIGHT CLASS

This was not my first experience coaching marathoners. A dozen years earlier, I had worked with Ron Gunn, dean of sports education at Southwestern Michigan College (SMC) in Dowagiac, Michigan, to teach adults how to finish a marathon. Dubbed the Monday Night Class because that was when we met, this was one of the first running classes designed for adult runners, as opposed to student-athletes.

Gunn coached track and cross-country at SMC, winning several national junior college championships. My son Kevin ran on one of those championship teams in 1978. Dowagiac was a small town of 6,583 located in Cass County, Michigan, which had the distinction of having more pig farms than any other county in the United States. The nickname for the college's sports teams was Roadrunners, and Gunn maintained a close relationship with the townspeople, who often came to meets to cheer his teams. The teams did their part by helping with local charitable projects.

Gunn also belonged to the Rotary Club, as did lumberyard operator Dick Judd, who told Gunn one evening: "You keep preaching how running is good for you. When are you going to teach us how to do it?"

At first, Gunn was not enthusiastic about organizing a jogging class. First, he was busy enough coaching his teams and supervising the athletic department. Second, he suspected that most of those who said they might join a jogging class would soon lose interest and move on to something else. He purposely scheduled the class on Monday night in competition with ABC's *Monday Night Football*, figuring that would hasten the class's demise.

Gunn underestimated his own ability to motivate adults as well as college students. The fact that Dowagiac was a small town where many in the class already knew one another from churches or clubs undoubtedly contributed to the easy sociability that developed. The class was divided evenly between men and women, many of them couples. Many of the men belonged to Rotary. Many of the women were members of the Junior Arts Club. A large number attended First Methodist Church.

Several members of his class lost as much as 100 pounds. Others were able to stop smoking. They discovered that although running was never easy, it was more fun than they had thought. Class members often ended runs at one another's houses, sticking around to chat and drink a beer or two. "Sociability became the key to maintaining interest," says Gunn. When the class finished one run at a local bar, the owner and his wife decided that the group was having so much fun, they too would enroll. A year later and 30 pounds lighter, the bar owners finished their first marathon.

"The best dating service in town."

That was when I got involved, working with Gunn to design a training program that would prepare a group of middle-aged men and women to complete a marathon. From my own successful distance-running career, I knew the type of training necessary for runners at the front of the pack to run fast times. I was not yet certain how you trained people to finish in the middle or even the back of the pack, particularly when those people had started running only a few weeks before. I would soon learn. In the second year of the program, Ron and I led a group of thirty-five runners to the Honolulu Marathon, and each one of them finished—and finished with smiles on their faces.

This was a rewarding time for me, as well as for members of the class. In retrospect, the training program I designed for that first Monday Night Class was much harsher, with much more mileage than I now feel is necessary for first-time marathoners, but it proved a beginning for me as a marathon coach. One important element, based on my own training and what I knew about the training of elite runners at that time, was the step-up, step-back approach similar to that used in St. Louis and other cities where innovative coaches guided marathon hopefuls. Like many teachers, I feel I learned as much from my students as they from me. The Monday Night Class continues to this day. Not everybody still runs marathons—or even runs—because many of the class's original members have switched from running to walking.

It is important to rest after the weekend long run.

Several years after training the Monday Night Class, I began coaching my son Kevin, who after two years at SMC transferred to Indiana University, graduating in 1982. Kevin wanted to qualify for the 1984 Olympic trials in the marathon. To do so, he would need to match the trials standard of 2:19:05, no easy task for someone who had a full-time job for a Big Eight accounting firm, Peat Marwick Mitchell. That plus a girlfriend, also a member of the firm, who eventually became his wife.

To efficiently use Kevin's time, I designed a training program that crammed most of the hard work—including a weekly long run—into the weekend, when he had more hours not only to train but also to rest from that hard training. I bracketed weekends of hard training, including long runs, with rest on Fridays and Mondays. Kevin eventually did achieve that trials qualifying time (2:18:50) at the 1983 Lake County Marathon, in the northern suburbs of Chicago.

THE CHICAGO PATTERN

Thus, when Brian Piper asked me to help train runners in the Chicago Marathon training class, I was able to draw on my experience coaching both the Monday Night Class and my son, Kevin. Over a period of time, Piper and I modified the training approach, expanding the time period from 15 to 18 weeks and also cutting back on the up-front mileage in recognition that not everybody joins the class with a 30- to 50-mile-a-week base. (That was something I had learned working with the Monday Night Class.) Blessed with youthful enthusiasm, many of the runners who joined our class had chosen the marathon as their first race, never having seen the starting line of a 5K. Like Kevin, they also had busy lives, so they did not always have time for midweek runs that lasted more than an hour—but they did have this time on the weekends.

What might be called the weekend Cram Course became key to the success of our program, but equally important was the step-back concept. Cutting the long run mileage back every third week allowed runners to recover both physically and psychologically for the next step up in mileage. Toward the end of the program, when long-run mileage approached its peak of 20 miles, we inserted step-back weeks every other week. By stretching less mileage over a slightly longer period, we found that we could reduce runners' risks of injury and increase their chances of success. At the same time, we also offered intermediate and advanced programs for runners seeking to improve on their previous marathon times. The intermediate programs offered more mileage; the advanced programs introduced speedwork.

The training program I developed for Chicago with Brian Piper's assistance followed this approach for novice runners.

Monday: No running. It is important to rest after the weekend long run.

Tuesday: Easy runs building from 3 miles to a maximum of 5 miles by Week 14 of the 18-week program. Tuesday (along with Thursday) is a good day to do some strength training, coupled with extra stretching.

Wednesday: The second-longest run of the week: 3 miles, building to 10 miles by Week 15. I call this my sorta-long day.

Thursday: The same as Tuesday: an easy run of 3 to 5 miles.

Friday: No running. It is important to rest before the weekend long run. All my programs—including those for intermediate and advanced runners—prescribe Friday as a day off from training.

Saturday: The key to the marathon program: a long run that builds from 6 miles in Week 1 to 20 miles in Week 15, but with step-backs every third week to permit runners to gather energy for the next push upward.

Sunday: Cross-training of about an hour for recovery. This could be cycling, swimming, walking, or even some light jogging. Runners who do their long runs on Sundays cross-train on Saturdays.

The maximum weekly mileage for my novice marathon training program is 40 miles in Week 15, when we do our 20-miler. In general, novice runners cover about as many miles during the rest of the week as they do in their long weekend run. (For instance, in Week 11, the long run is 16 miles; the total mileage that week is 32.) Intermediate and advanced runners do somewhat more mileage as they strive for improved times.

What I now identify as my Novice 1 training program (page 324) follows a simple schedule, but it works—as thousands of runners have proved. In fact, tens of thousands, perhaps hundreds of thousands, of runners follow this same schedule, which is posted on my website and is also available in an interactive format through TrainingPeaks. Although technology has made it possible to offer my marathon training programs in a variety of ways, running can still be as simple as you want to make it. You start out in Week 1 with a run of a few miles; you finish in Week 18 triumphantly crossing the finish line of a 26-mile-385-yard race.

Piper warns: "Running a marathon never will be easy. If it were easy, the challenge would be gone. But learning to train right can increase your enjoyment in both training for and running the race."

11

Moving Beyond 26.2

The Ultramarathon

Just because you crossed the finish line in your first precisely measured 26-mile-385-yard race, it's not yet time to join Peggy Lee
in asking, "Is that all there is?" There definitely is more, and the
"more" is called the ultramarathon.

An *ultramarathon* (aka *ultra*) is any running race longer than 26.2 miles
or 42.2 kilometers. For many, if not most, nouveau ultramarathoners,
the next and logical step upward in distance is 50 kilometers, 50K, or
31.1 miles. A 50K is 5 miles longer than the standard marathon you
may just have finished. It's a much larger jump to the next round number, 50 miles (80.5 kilometers), but I have provided training programs
for both the 50K and the 50-mile at the end of this chapter. The next
rounded-off jump after that? One hundred miles. That takes a huge
leap of faith: not quite climbing Mount Everest, but moving in the same
direction.

Not all ultramarathons come rounded off. The world's largest, oldest,
and most prestigious ultra is the Comrades Marathon between Durban
and Pietermaritzburg in South Africa. I use the word *between* because the

race changes directions every year. Five massive hills separate Durban on the ocean from Pietermaritzburg inland. Heading to Pietermaritzburg, you go "up." Return the following year, and you go "down," although downhill miles are not easier than uphill miles unless you have trained your quadriceps muscles to resist the pounding. Because of the shifts in direction, the race distance fluctuates somewhere around 55 miles, or 89 kilometers. That seems appropriate, since for many ultramarathoners, it is not about distance, it is about meeting a challenge (like climbing Everest). The Comrades organizers don't seem to worry about exact distances either, and why should they? Founded in 1921 in memory of South African soldiers killed in World War I, Comrades attracts twenty-five thousand runners each year; incredibly, entries are limited to that number. Comrades is like Boston in that there is a stiff qualifying standard. Boston has its BQ for *Boston qualifier*; Comrades has its CQ for *Comrades qualifier.* To get into this most ultra of all ultramarathons, runners must qualify by finishing an officially recognized marathon faster than 4 hours 50 minutes, that being the 2019 standard.

But most ultramarathons (as many as 80 percent, suggests Cory Smith of *UltraRunning* magazine) are run not on pavement but on trails that cut through the woods and onto desert sands, and even across rocky mountain ranges. Jason Daley ranked "The 9 Toughest Ultramarathons" in an article for *Outside* magazine, the toughest of the tough being the Marathon des Sables, a 6-day, 154-mile trek through the Sahara Desert in southern Morocco. Also on the *Outside* list was the Hardrock 100, which includes 33,992 feet of ascent and descent on its mountain course near Silverton, Colorado. Daley wrote: "Being above treeline for most of the course, racers are also vulnerable to lightning and freak storms."

Despite the challenge offered by these extralong races, despite the extra miles seemingly needed both for training and for racing, participation in these longest of long-distance races seems to be in an uptick, at least based on runners signing up for my 50K program on the Internet: nearly a 30 percent increase between 2018 and 2019. *UltraRunning* magazine reports 2,129 races and 115,693 finishers in 2018. Two out of every three competitors are male.

A HISTORY OF ULTRAS

Those numbers seem stunning. Fifty years ago, you could count the number of 26-mile marathons in North America on the fingers of one hand. There was Boston, of course, the world's oldest marathon, and Yonkers in New York and Culver City out in California and another marathon up in Canada, Saint-Hyacinthe. Maybe one or two others. One hundred fifty-one runners ran Boston in 1959, my first year running. No qualifying standard needed, and the entry fee was $1. Ultramarathons? You've got to be kidding. *UltraRunning* publisher Karl Hoagland identifies the JFK 50 Mile, started in 1963, as the oldest North American ultra. The race is still going strong with one thousand entrants a year. America's finest ultramarathoner back in that era was Olympian Ted Corbitt, but he needed to travel to England to find a 26-plus race worthy of his talents. In 1965, I went to London on assignment from *Sports Illustrated* to report on Ted running the London to Brighton marathon, the world's second most prestigious ultra at that time, second only to Comrades. Ted finished second. My article on that achievement eventually appeared in the second issue of a newly established running publication, *Distance Running News*, later to be renamed *Runner's World*.

Nobody could have predicted how big ultramarathon running would become, doubling in the last decade. Hoagland believes part of the attraction is that "after you have done X number of marathons, the next logical step is an ultra."

The training is tougher, the racing is tougher, but Hoagland points to the community spirit at ultramarathons, where people compete with themselves and with each other to overcome audacious, sometimes life-changing challenges. "In this troubled world," Hoagland says, "ultramarathons have become a sanctuary from the storm by providing an epic experience in a positive and supportive environment that explores and celebrates the outer bounds of human potential. And it's not just the racers, since the volunteers, crew, and pacers at 100-mile races put as much into the events as the runners. But they do so in some of the most scenic settings in the world."

Adila Khazali of Kuala Lumpur agrees: "Ultras are a serious game-changer. For anyone who feels that their running game is boring these days, train for and run an ultra. It sounds crazy, but it'll give you the experience of a lifetime."

AND THEN THE VULTURE EATS YOU

Among my 111 marathons, may I confess, only two were run at distances beyond 26.2. Both my ultras, separated by several decades, were in South Africa. I ran well in the first, a 50K at altitude between Johannesburg and Pietermaritzburg. The second, Comrades, humbled me in that I failed to make the cut-off time that would have earned me a medal. A more important ultra on my curriculum vitae is the Trans-Indiana Run, a one-time event (not a "race") that my running buddy Steve Kearney and I organized one summer almost as a lark, recruiting a total of ten participants mainly by word of mouth. Trans-Indiana covered the length of the state of Indiana "from river to shining lake," the Ohio River to Lake Michigan, 350 miles in 10 days. I learned several important lessons during that run, held midsummer with temperatures in the 80s and 90s: (1) Proper (and specialized) training is essential; and (2) the vulture definitely will eat you if you fail to master your nutritional needs not only in the event but during the months of training leading up to the event.

Later, while researching this chapter, I wondered what training tips or tricks separated ultramarathoners from marathoners. What do ultramarathoners know that we shorter-distance runners have not yet discovered and perhaps never will? I decided to pose the question to my followers on Twitter. These were the strategies that I felt were most important:

1. More miles training
2. Good training program
3. Proper pacing
4. Nutrition before and during

The results of my Twitter poll were surprising (see the sidebar) in that only two percentage points separated all four strategies. The proper answer to my polled question appeared to be "all of the above."

SECRETS OF SUCCESS

Ultramarathoners told me what contributed most to their success:

1. More miles training	24%
2. Good training program	25%
3. Proper pacing	26%
4. Nutrition before and during	25%

FOUR TIPS FOR ULTRAMARATHONERS

Let's consider each of the four strategies:

1. MORE MILES TRAINING

When Ted Corbitt trained for ultramarathons, he often ran daily from his home near Van Cortlandt Park to his work (as a physical therapist) in Midtown Manhattan, 20 miles one way in the morning, 12 miles home on a slightly different course in the evening. This caused one individual hanging out on a corner whom Ted passed regularly to say, "Man, that cat's late to work every morning." Few runners I knew could have matched Ted Corbitt's training mileages. During Labor Day weekend, while preparing for London to Brighton, Ted circled Manhattan Island (31 miles), then kept going on a second lap (62 miles total). But that was only Saturday! He then repeated that route on Sunday and Monday for a grand weekend total of 186 miles. On several occasions, according to his son Gary, Ted ran more than 300 miles in a single 7-day week.

But most of us are mortals, and that includes Angel Diaz of New Jersey, who followed one of my training programs for his first 50K in Philadelphia. A busy work schedule sometimes forced him to miss some runs, but not the most important runs: "I made sure I did my long runs no matter what. Aside from being honest about my training it was mainly becoming mentally strong." So, "more miles training" does count.

2. GOOD TRAINING PROGRAM

Ultramarathoner Garrick Arends of Meridian, Idaho, favors quality training over high mileage. It is not entirely how many miles you run, Arends explains, but more how you run those miles. This was true with Steve Kearney and me as we prepared for Trans-Indiana. We did our long runs (plural) on two or more consecutive days, not just a single day. To that point, we might do a 2-hour run on Saturday followed by a 5-hour run on Sunday, running mostly on trails in Indiana Dunes State Park, not caring how much distance we covered, simply getting out and spending time on our feet. During the week, we ran fewer miles at slower paces so we would not arrive at the weekend too tired to train.

I recycled Trans-Indiana when I designed the 50K training program at the end of this chapter. Many ultramarathoners ignore distance, focusing on however long it takes to finish whatever distance they covered. For this reason, training for an ultramarathon is not necessarily tougher than training for a regular marathon. You get to pause for a drink without worrying that you are losing time. Racing an ultramarathon also may not necessarily be tougher than racing 26.2 if you heed the advice in the next paragraph.

3. PROPER PACING

I opened this book with the quick tip I often offered runners at expos the day before their marathons: "Start slow." That sounds oh so simple, but it isn't really. You need to *control* your pace, as Dan Lyne of Camas, Washington, explains: "It is essential that you learn how to run slow. If you're only running 10 to 13 miles in a workout, it may seem you're running *too slow*, but you'll find out differently when you stretch those distances to 26, particularly in an ultra."

Here's a plus. Since most ultras, particularly the longest ultras on trails, are run at slower paces than marathons, you will lose less time if you shift, now and then, from run pace to walk pace—or even walk for long periods. Important: Don't shift to walking pace only in races. Practice walking pace, and particularly practice shifting back and forth from walking to running pace. Don't leave your run-walk-run strategies to chance.

4. NUTRITION BEFORE AND DURING

In speaking about marathon nutrition, keep in mind two words: *Carbs rule!* Fast-forward, if you please, to page 212: "The Distance Runner's Diet." A proper diet for long-distance runners, I will explain, contains ample amounts of carbohydrate.

But...

And it's a very big *but*. Not everybody agrees. Popular among ultramarathoners is the ketogenic diet, a diet high in fat (70 percent); somewhat high in protein (20 percent); but almost devoid of carbohydrates (10 percent). In contrast, I recommend a diet high in carbohydrates (55 percent) ahead of fats (30 percent) and proteins (15 percent). That's the so-called Golden Standard, the diet I have followed most of my life.

Here's the theory behind the keto diet: The body burns carbohydrates, which it turns into glycogen, quite efficiently. It is your rocket fuel. But if you limit carb intake while training for an ultra, you force your body to turn to fats for fuel. Burning fat requires more oxygen than burning carbohydrates. This "teaches" the body to more efficiently burn fats. Thus, in the 99th mile of a 100-miler, after the quickly burned carbohydrates have been consumed, keto supporters believe that the fats remain to speed you to the finish line.

However, in discussions with nutritionists, most specifically Nancy Clark, RD, author of *Nancy Clark's Sports Nutrition Guidebook* and a fellow of both the Academy of Nutrition and Dietetics and the ACSM, I haven't come across any believable, scientific proof favoring fats over carbs, specifically for competitive athletes who train at high intensity. Nevertheless, among some experienced ultramarathoners, fats do rule. And if you have diabetes, the dietary rules for you are much different. If after a few marathons you want to experiment with a keto lifestyle, give it a try. Clark writes: "Each athlete needs to learn through trial and error during training and competition what works best for his or her body and what doesn't work."

ULTRAMARATHON: 50K

Training for a 50K race is only slightly different than training for a 26-mile race. Unlike in my standard, 18-week programs, every other weekly long run is time-based rather than mileage-based. This is for psychological as much as for physical reasons. Three or more hours of running somehow sounds much more manageable than a specific distance. Since 80 percent of ultramarathons are run on trails rather than pavement, you need not know how far you ran (or walked) in any specific workout. One quick explanation concerning the difference between a "run" and a "pace" run. A run can be done at any speed, depending on how you feel that day; a run at "pace," more specifically "race pace," is a run done at the precise pace you want to hit in your goal race.

Week	Mon	Tue	Wed	Thu	Fri	Sat	Sun
1	Rest	3-mile run	5-mile run	3-mile run	Rest	5-mile pace	10-mile run
2	Rest	3-mile run	5-mile run	3-mile run	Rest	5-mile run	1.5-hour run
3	Rest	3-mile run	6-mile run	3-mile run	Rest	6-mile pace	8-mile run
4	Rest	3-mile run	6-mile run	3-mile run	Rest	6-mile pace	13-mile run
5	Rest	3-mile run	7-mile run	3-mile run	Rest	7-mile run	2-hour run
6	Rest	3-mile run	7-mile run	3-mile run	Rest	7-mile pace	10-mile run
7	Rest	4-mile run	8-mile run	4-mile run	Rest	5-mile pace	16-mile run
8	Rest	4-mile run	8-mile run	4-mile run	Rest	8-mile run	2.5-hour run
9	Rest	4-mile run	9-mile run	4-mile run	Rest	Rest	13.1-mile run
10	Rest	4-mile run	9-mile run	4-mile run	Rest	9-mile pace	3-hour run
11	Rest	5-mile run	10-mile run	5-mile run	Rest	10-mile run	20-mile run
12	Rest	5-mile run	6-mile run	5-mile run	Rest	6-mile pace	2-hour run
13	Rest	5-mile run	10-mile run	5-mile run	Rest	10-mile pace	20-mile run
14	Rest	5-mile run	6-mile run	5-mile run	Rest	6-mile run	2.5-hour run
15	Rest	5-mile run	10-mile run	5-mile run	Rest	10-mile pace	20-mile run
16	Rest	5-mile run	8-mile run	5-mile run	Rest	10-mile pace	3-hour run
17	Rest	4-mile run	6-mile run	4-mile run	Rest	4-mile pace	8-mile run
18	Rest	3-mile run	4-mile	Rest	Rest	2-mile run	26-mile run
19	Rest	Rest	Rest	3-mile run	Rest	1-hour run	1-hour run
20	Rest	3-mile run	10-mile run	3-mile run	Rest	1-hour pace	3-hour run

(continued)

21	Rest	3-mile run	6-mile run	3-mile run	Rest	1.5-hour run	2-hour run
22	Rest	3-mile run	10-mile run	3-mile run	Rest	1.5-hour pace	4-hour run
23	Rest	4-mile run	7-mile run	4-mile run	Rest	2-hour run	3-hour run
24	Rest	4-mile run	10-mile run	4-mile run	Rest	2-hour pace	5-hour pace
25	Rest	4-mile run	8-mile run	4-mile run	Rest	1-hour run	1-hour run
26	Rest	4-mile run	4-mile run	Rest	Rest	2-mile run	31.1-mile run

ULTRAMARATHON: 50 MILES

Nobody said making the jump from 50 kilometers to 50 miles was easy, but running ultramarathons is never easy, otherwise the challenge would not appeal to so many runners for whom 26.2 is not enough. To train for 50 miles, simply add the following 8 weeks of training to the 26-week 50K program. Note also that the 50-mile program suggests time-based training on both Saturdays and Sundays.

27	Rest	Rest	Rest	4-mile run	Rest	1-hour run	2-hour run
28	Rest	5-mile run	10-mile run	5-mile run	Rest	1.5-hour run	3-hour run
29	Rest	5-mile run	8-mile run	5-mile run	Rest	2-hour pace	4-hour run
30	Rest	5-mile run	10-mile run	5-mile run	Rest	2.5-hour run	5-hour run
31	Rest	6-mile run	8-mile run	6-mile run	Rest	2.5-hour pace	6-hour run
32	Rest	6-mile run	10-mile run	6-mile run	Rest	3-hour run	3-hour run
33	Rest	5-mile run	8-mile run	5-mile run	Rest	2-hour pace	2-hour run
34	Rest	4-mile run	6-mile run	Rest	Rest	2-mile run	50-mile run

THE DOPEY CHALLENGE

Truth be told, the Dopey Challenge is not an ultramarathon, except in total miles run over four consecutive days at Walt Disney World: 5K on Thursday, 10K on Friday, a half marathon on Saturday and, finally, a full marathon on Sunday, close to 50 miles total. Yes, I suppose you have to be "dopey" to accept that challenge, but Dopey has proved increasingly popular among runners who also visit theme parks with their families between runs. The key to this program is to gradually, during a standard 18-week buildup, adapt your body to running on consecutive days. And (most important), don't run so fast on the first few days and arrive at the fourth day with your energy stores drained. In addition to Dopey, a number of road relays (Hood to Coast in Oregon being the most popular) entice competitors to run multiple legs on multiple days. This Dopey training program can serve as a pattern for such races. Week 1 offers a 13-miler. Does that seem far for you? If so, maybe you are not Dopey enough to accept this challenge.

Week	Mon	Tue	Wed	Thu	Fri	Sat	Sun
1	Rest	3-mile run	5-mile pace	3-mile run	Rest	3-mile run	13-mile run
2	Rest	3-mile run	5-mile run	3-mile run	Rest	7-mile run	Cross
3	Rest	3-mile run	5-mile pace	3-mile run	Rest	4-mile run	14-mile run
4	Rest	3-mile run	6-mile pace	3-mile run	Rest	8-mile run	Cross
5	Rest	3-mile run	6-mile run	3-mile run	Rest	5-mile run	15-mile run
6	Rest	3-mile run	6-mile pace	3-mile run	Rest	9-mile run	Cross
7	Rest	4-mile run	7-mile pace	4-mile run	Rest	6-mile run	16-mile run

(continued)

8	Rest	4-mile run	7-mile run	4-mile run	Rest	10-mile run	Cross
9	Rest	4-mile run	7-mile pace	Rest	2-mile run	7-mile run	17-mile run
10	Rest	4-mile run	8-mile pace	4-mile run	Rest	11-mile run	Cross
11	Rest	5-mile run	8-mile run	Rest	3-mile run	8-mile run	18-mile run
12	Rest	5-mile run	8-mile pace	5-mile run	Rest	12-mile run	Cross
13	Rest	5-mile run	5-mile pace	Rest	4-mile run	9-mile run	19-mile run
14	Rest	5-mile run	8-mile run	5-mile run	Rest	13-mile run	Cross
15	Rest	5-mile run	Rest	2.5-mile run	5-mile run	10-mile run	20-mile run
16	Rest	5-mile run	Rest	4-mile run	Rest	12-mile run	Cross
17	Rest	4-mile run	Rest	3-mile run	Rest	8-mile run	Cross
18	Rest	2-mile run	Rest	5K	10K	Half	Marathon

12

Speedwork

If You Want to Run Fast,
You Need to Run Fast

Speedwork! That's a scary word, a frightening concept to a lot of marathoners, who reason that there is nothing speedy about the pace at which they run 26-mile races. If that is so, why do speedwork, with its apparent threat of injury? Most marathoners want to run far, not fast. One runner who picked up a copy of my book with that title (*Run Fast*) at a race expo where I was signing copies grunted, "I don't want to run fast." Fair enough. If you are a marathoner, you probably need to do speedwork only if you want to improve your performance.

Did that get your attention? If so, let's consider some of the ways marathoners can benefit by doing speedwork.

First, speedwork is an effective means for improvement—even for marathoners. Coupled with endurance training, speedwork can get you to almost any goal. According to Alfred F. Morris, PhD, a health and fitness manager from Washington, D.C., "It is important for runners to learn to run fast so that the marathon pace feels comfortable." Adds Frank X. Mari, a coach from Toms River, New Jersey: "You will never see full potential as a marathon runner until you develop your full potential as a sprinter." Coach Keith Woodard of Portland, Oregon, adds: "You have to be able to run fast at short distances before you can run fast at long distances." But, one caveat: As mentioned in earlier chapters, first-time marathoners need give little attention to speedwork. Their main goal is to gradually (and gently) increase their mileage so that they can finish a 26-mile race. Improving marathoners probably should also focus their attention on determining what level of high-mileage training works best for them. But after you have been running for several years and begin to shave seconds instead of minutes off your PRs, or if you start to slip backward, it is time to turn to speedwork.

SPEED LIMITS

Speedwork seems scary to many—but maybe not as much as people think. In an Internet survey, I asked runners, "Do you do speedwork?" Three out of four claimed that they sometimes do; another 14 percent claimed that they speed train all the time. Only one out of ten have never tried speedwork and probably are quite happy keeping it that way.

DO YOU DO SPEEDWORK?

Never have done speedwork	8%
May some day do speedwork	12%
Speed train some of the time	66%
Speed train all of the time	14%

SPEEDWORK BENEFITS

Although long-distance runners concede that speedwork forms an integral part of any well-designed training regimen, not all marathoners use it as part of their training. One reason is unfamiliarity. Many of today's adult runners did not compete in track or on cross-country teams in high school or college, so speedwork and running tracks feel foreign to them.

There is also an element of fear, both of the unknown and of injury—with good reason, since by training at too high an intensity, you can hurt yourself. (Notice I said "too high." We'll come to that later.)

Admittedly, speedwork can hurt, and the burning sensation you get in your lungs and the ache in your legs may seem more threatening than the less piercing fatigue you encounter running the roads. Usually after a hard workout on the track, particularly early in the season, your legs will remain sore for several days. (I hope you have your massage therapist on speed dial.)

You will perform better at all distances and levels.

Also, you cannot hold a decent conversation while zipping through a speed session. As for wearing a music-playing device, after a few fast sessions on the track, you probably will discard that device, at least until your cooldown laps. There's a simple reason for this: To do speedwork properly, you need to concentrate intently, and listening to music poses an unneeded distraction. Nevertheless, there are ten good reasons every long-distance runner should do speedwork on a track.

1. PERFORMANCE

This is the most valid reason. With speedwork, you will run faster. That is guaranteed. Numerous laboratory studies have proved that adding speed training to an endurance base can take seconds off 5K times and minutes off marathon bests. Melvin H. Williams, PhD, of the Human Performance Laboratory at Old Dominion University, once told me: "By training faster, you improve specific muscles used at higher speeds. You also improve your anaerobic threshold, which allows you to run a faster pace and remain aerobic. If you can run faster at short distances, you can increase your absolute ability at longer distances, too."

2. FORM

One of the most effective ways I know—in fact, the best way—to improve form is by running fast in practice. If you can learn to run more efficiently (exercise physiologists prefer the term *economically*), you will perform better at all distances and levels. I am not sure why speed training improves your running form. Maybe you recruit different muscles. Maybe you force yourself to move more smoothly. Maybe by learning how to run at speeds faster than race pace, you become more relaxed when you do run race pace in a marathon. Maybe it is all of these reasons. Whatever the reason, running fast works.

3. VARIETY

Running the same course and the same distance at the same pace day after day after day can become tedious. To keep running exciting, you need variety. Many road-running clubs organize weekly speed sessions as a benefit to their members. When my wife and I stayed at our Florida condo during the winter, I often would train with the group that meets Wednesday evenings at the Bolles School track in Jacksonville. I would go there as much for social reasons as to improve my speed, but I noticed that many of my training companions took their Wednesday night track workouts *very* seriously.

4. EXCITEMENT

Running alone through scenic trails provides its own pleasure, but tracks can have a level of activity that can stimulate you during your workouts. During my early career, I trained frequently at Stagg Field on the campus of the University of Chicago. (I competed many years for the University of Chicago Track Club, organized by the school's coach, also an Olympic coach, Ted Haydon.) There always seemed to be half a dozen activities going on simultaneously: rugby in the infield, tennis behind the stands, several softball games on an adjoining field, kids playing in the sand of the long-jump pit, and track athletes practicing multiple events. There was an electricity in this whirlwind of athletic activity that I found enormously appealing.

5. CONVENIENCE

There are tracks in every city and town, so it is very convenient to find one where you can do your workouts. Another important point: You can obtain maximum benefit in minimum time by doing speedwork. Here's a workout Olympian Fred Wilt, one of my former coaches, taught me: Head to the track and run eight laps, which is 2 miles (3200 meters). Run the first four laps (1600 meters) at a comfortable warmup pace. Then, without stopping, run the next 200 meters hard and the following 200 easy, and repeat this pattern once more for a total of four more laps (eight laps total for the workout). You are done, and your workout will have taken only about 20 minutes. That interval workout would be expressed as 4 × 200 (200 jog). The final 200 jog serves as your cooldown, and then you're in the car, heading home for dinner. (The same workout—once you learn the pattern—can be done on the road or on trails as well as on a track.)

6. CONCENTRATION

One skill that separates the good runners from the almost-good runners is an ability to focus their attention for the entire period of the race, whether it is a mile or a marathon. Dissociating is a good strategy for beginning marathoners, but not for people who want to run fast. When your mind wanders during a marathon, inevitably you slow down. If you stay focused, you learn how to concentrate all body systems to sustain a steady pace, conserve your energy, and maintain your running form. It takes total concentration to run fast on a track; once you master this skill, you can transfer it to your road runs.

7. SAFETY

You cannot get hit by a car while running on a track, and you probably will not be chased by a dog, either. If you are in the company of others, the danger of being mugged is reduced. On a hot or cold day, if you become overheated or chilled or fatigued, you can just walk off the track and head for your car or the locker room; you do not have to worry about being caught 3 miles from home and trudging those final miles at a diminishing pace. Also, there are usually drinking fountains and toilets nearby at running tracks.

8. COMPANIONSHIP

Willie Sutton was once asked why he robbed banks, and his response was, "Because that's where the money is." Well, tracks are where the runners are. On a track, you can seek company and training partners, and partners are important if you want to run fast. It sometimes becomes difficult to motivate yourself to train hard when you are alone. With someone running those interval quarters with you, you may get a better workout and improve. But beware: A companion danger is that you may train too hard, resulting in staleness (aka *burnout*) or injury. On balance, however, your running will improve if you find running partners with whom you enjoy training.

Whatever the reason, running fast works.

9. MOTIVATION

Your running also will improve if you can find a coach to guide you in your training. A second variation of the Willie Sutton rule is that you find coaches at tracks. Because it is difficult to watch runners and monitor their strengths and weaknesses when they are scattered all over a road, most coaches prefer to gather people in groups for speedwork sessions. My grandson Kyle Higdon ran cross-country at Notre Dame, then coached a club team while attending graduate school at the University of Texas at Austin. They met weekly, one of Kyle's favorite workouts being running repeats around the Texas State Capitol building, each lap about a half mile. Probably the single most important asset a coach can offer a runner is motivation. Any runner can select one of the many training programs offered in this book or on the Internet, but a skilled coach can motivate you and guide you to follow that program properly.

10. PLEASURE

Just as it feels good for a tennis player to hit the ball perfectly over the net or for a golfer to loft a well-aimed chip shot to the green, it also feels good to run fast. There is a certain tactile pleasure in doing any activity well, an experience that in running I call "feeling the wind in your hair." One way to achieve the pleasure of fast running is to run short distances interspersed with adequate periods of rest—in other words, speedwork. And because speedwork inevitably will help you improve your performance on race day, that boost will add to your pleasure, too.

DEFINING SPEEDWORK

I define speedwork in *Run Fast* as "any training done at race pace or faster." In that book, I offered advice for runners seeking to improve their 5K and 10K times, so I related race pace to how fast they ran those distances. In other words, race pace changes depending on the distance of the race for which you are preparing. If you run the marathon in 4:30, you run at a pace of 10:18 per mile, but to go out and run half a dozen miles at your marathon pace—which most experienced runners could achieve easily—would not necessarily constitute speedwork. Speed-work for marathoners is training done at a pace significantly faster than they would run in a marathon. Your 10K pace still remains an excellent benchmark.

To further define speedwork, I probably should add that it usually involves bursts of fast running (at or faster than race pace) followed by periods of slower running, or rest, the so-called interval in interval training.

When your mind wanders during a marathon, inevitably you slow down.

That's essential because most runners probably can achieve race pace for long distances only when motivated and well rested—in other words, during the race itself. To achieve race pace in practice, they need to cut their race distance into segments and rest between those segments. If you were a competitor at 5000 meters, you could run 12 × 400 meters in a workout, resting for short periods after each 400, and simulate some of the stress of your race while practicing race pace. A marathon runner probably would not do 26 × mile in a single workout, but the principle remains the same.

There are different ways to do speedwork. Some work better for marathoners than for runners competing at shorter distances. You can run repeats, intervals, sprints, strides, surges, fartlek, or tempo runs (terms I am about to define). You can run these workouts on the track, down the road, or on a path in the woods. And for weather-challenged runners, you can run on a treadmill in a gym. You do not even need a measured distance and a stopwatch; you can measure intensity by using a pulse monitor or even perceived exertion. And now we have Global Positioning System (GPS) watches and apps that track the length of your fast burst with reasonable precision. In *Run Fast*, I devote a chapter to each of the speedwork variations, describing them in detail. In summary, here are the various types of speedwork and their applicability to marathon training.

REPEATS

In a repeat workout, you run very fast, usually over a very short distance, and take a relatively long period of time to recover before repeating that distance. The fast (or hard) run in repeats is referred to as a *repetition*, or a *rep*. The runner recovers almost fully between reps, either jogging or completely resting. When I coached high school distance runners, I often had them walk a timed 5 minutes between reps. That allowed them to recover sufficiently so they could run

> **It feels good to run fast.**

each rep at near maximum speed. There's nothing magic about 5 minutes, but resting for that precise amount of time at each workout offered them a familiar benchmark.

LONG REPEATS

Most marathon coaches believe runners should do their long runs slower than race pace. To do otherwise is to risk injury. Yet they agree on the need to do *some* running at the pace you plan to run your marathon so you can familiarize both your mind and muscles with that pace. So when and how do you run race pace?

The answer is long repeats.

Just as milers go to the track and do interval workouts of 10 × 400 or 16 × 200 at a fast pace, jogging or walking in between each rep for recovery, experienced marathoners can do long repeats as a form of speed training. Runners training for 5K and 10K races can also benefit from long repeats, although this workout is not advised for first-time marathoners. Long repeats are best done on the roads on a course featuring mile markers. If there is no such course nearby, you can always use a GPS watch to make

(continued)

measurements. Good distances for long repeat workouts are the half-mile, mile, 1.5-mile, and 2-mile. Run one of those distances at race pace once, rest for 2 to 3 minutes by walking and/or jogging slowly, and then repeat. Over a period of weeks and months, you can gradually increase the number of repeats, but you should always run race pace because familiarization is one of the most important reasons for this workout.

Here are several patterns for runners training for different race distances. Over a period of weeks and months, begin at the lower numbers and increase to the higher numbers.

Goal Race	Starting Workout	Goal Workout
5K	3 × half-mile	6 × half-mile
10K	3 × mile	6 × mile
Half marathon	2 × 1.5-mile	5 × 1.5-mile
Marathon	2 × 2-mile	5 × 2-mile

Taper the workout 2 to 3 weeks before your important race. If your goal is not a specific race, you can vary your training by alternating between different repeat distances week to week. Or if your goal is a fast marathon, begin with the 5K repeat distances and gradually progress to those for the marathon.

INTERVALS

In interval training, you carefully control the period of rest time, or interval, between the fast repetitions. Usually there are more reps than in repeat workouts, and the distance (or time) of the interval between fast reps is shorter. Key to this kind of workout is that your heart rate not be allowed to drop too low before you surge into action again. Please note that the interval is the period between reps, not the repetition itself. Interval training is a more stressful form of training than most other forms of speedwork because you are never quite allowed to relax, so the result is a steady buildup of fatigue. For this reason, many veteran long-distance runners shy away from this type of speedwork. On the other hand, interval training is probably the most efficient workout for developing speed. I titled my chapter on interval training in *Run Fast* "The Magic Workout"— quite accurately so, I might say.

SPRINTS

A sprint is just that: an all-out run for a short distance. The maximum distance a runner can do at full speed is probably around 300 meters, and that is only if the runner is extremely well trained. Most sprints run by distance runners in practice are probably shorter than that: 50 to 100 meters, a straightaway on a running track or a short fairway on a golf course. The object of running sprints in training is to develop style as well as speed, economy more than endurance. It is also a good way to stretch muscles and learn to lengthen your stride.

Why should marathon runners run sprints, when at no time during the race will they run anywhere near that speed? The reason is that sprints develop speed, and speed is basic to success in running, regardless of the distance. If you can develop your base speed at distances of 100 meters to a mile, inevitably you will become a faster marathon runner.

STRIDES

Strides are simply slow sprints. I frequently use strides as part of my warmup to get ready for a faster workout or before a race. Typically, I might jog a mile or two, stretch, then do 4 × 100 meters near race pace. Or I'll sometimes do strides at the end of a workout. Or, on a "rest" day, I'll do an easy workout that consists mainly of stretching and a few strides. Particularly during the summer months, I like to do these stride workouts barefoot on the fairway of a golf course in the early morning before the golfers appear.

I like to do strides at race pace regardless of the goal race distance, be it 800 meters or the marathon. Doing so reminds me of how fast I plan to race. The day before a marathon, I usually jog a mile or so for a warmup, pick a grassy place where I can run three or four easy strides at marathon pace, then jog a mile or so for a cooldown. It relaxes me for the race the next day. And on race day, I may do a couple of warmup strides, although as marathon fields grow in size to near forty thousand, it is often hard to warm up because of the crush of numbers.

SURGES

Surges are fast sprints thrown into the middle of a long run or a long race. Well, not too long a race. You probably should not surge too frequently in a marathon or you'll surge yourself into the pickup bus for runners who cannot finish. Although surging at the right time might win you an Olympic gold medal (as Joan Benoit proved in 1984), it is probably not a good race strategy for midpack runners, whose goal is to spread their energy evenly throughout the race to maximize performance. Nevertheless, surging is an effective and enjoyable training strategy. Surging is also one way to get yourself out of those "bad patches" that develop in the middle of even the best-trained runners' marathons. Sometimes a surge to a slightly faster pace allows you to recover as much as if you jogged along slowly.

> **Sprints develop speed, and speed is basic to success in running, regardless of the distance.**

FARTLEK

Fartlek is all of the above thrown into a single workout, usually done away from the track, preferably in the woods. It is a Swedish word that roughly translates to "speed play." Fartlek includes fast and slow running—maybe even walking. Basically, you jog or sprint or stride as the mood strikes you, alternating fast and slow running. One of my favorite T-shirts was one I saw worn by a woman in a race. On the front of the shirt was *Fartlek*. On the back of the shirt it said, *It's a runner's thing*.

Although fartlek is best practiced on wooded trails, marathoners can adapt this type of workout to their own needs on the roads. This is an unstructured form of speed training that appeals particularly to experienced runners who have become very adept at reading their body's signals and thus do not need the discipline of a stopwatch and a measured distance.

TEMPO RUNS

Exercise scientists now tell us that doing tempo runs is the most efficient way to raise your lactate threshold—that is, your ability to run at a fast pace without accumulating lactic acid in the bloodstream, which eventually will bring you to a halt. You train at the theoretical point between aerobic and anaerobic running.

I define tempo runs differently than do some coaches, who call any fast run at a steady pace "tempo." In my playbook, a tempo run is one in which you begin at an easy jogging pace, gradually accelerate to near your 10K race pace, hold that pace for several minutes, then gradually decelerate to your earlier jogging pace. A 40-minute tempo run might follow a pattern like this: Jog for 10 minutes, accelerate for 10 minutes, hold

> **"Fartlek. It's a runner's thing."**

near 10K pace for 10 minutes, decelerate for 10 minutes. There is nothing magic in the pattern of 10 + 10 + 10 + 10 = 40. A tempo run can follow any pattern, as long as you take yourself up to near the edge of your lactate threshold.

I find tempo runs done in this humpbacked fashion to be not only the most effective form of speedwork but also the most enjoyable. I love to do tempo runs on the trails of Indiana Dunes State Park near Chesterton, Indiana, about a 20-minute drive from my home. The surface of Trail 2 circling the marsh near Wilson Shelter is smooth, flat, and conducive to very fast running. Maybe it is partly the scenery (I often spot deer in the woods), but I usually finish my tempo runs invigorated and ready to beat the world.

All forms of speedwork can make you a better runner and a better marathoner. If you want to improve at any level of running, you have to learn to run fast.

SPEED FREAKS

When first-time marathoners ask if they should do speedwork, I answer no. If you have not done fast running before embarking on your marathon quest, this is no time to start. And unless you are following one of my advanced programs, which offer 1 or 2 days a week of speedwork, you are better off reserving this variety of training for what might be called the off-season.

Nevertheless, even though so-called experts warn that speedwork can increase the risk of injury (not always true if you do it right), most runners seeking improved performance do head to the track now and then. In one Internet survey I took for an earlier edition of this book, 86.4 percent of respondents confessed to being speed freaks. This was almost identical to the 87.5 percent response to the same survey done a half-dozen years earlier for the previous edition of this book.

Some comments by responders are worth sharing.

Meredith Caballero, Wichita Falls, Texas: "Speed training seems to not only help my times overall, but it breaks up the monotony of my running schedule. I usually have at least one speed session a week."

Martin Van Walsum, Carlisle, Massachusetts: "I never would have approached my capability if speedwork—runs at 5K or 10K pace—had not been part of my marathon training. A better term might be 'up tempo' running. The risk of injury is less at those paces, but the benefit in terms of stamina and strength is high."

Seth Harrison, Irvington, New York: "Speedwork for me consists of everything from a weekly fast-paced tempo run to longer runs at marathon pace. I don't speed train often, but without these workouts, my marathon times would be substantially slower."

Michele Keane, Atlanta, Georgia: "I love speedwork, but I'm a former track runner and enjoy the feeling of running fast. I incorporate fartlek, hills, and tempo runs in my training. I do know that as I age, I need to be smarter about how fast I run and how much I do."

Liz Reichman, San Antonio, Texas: "I speed train for two reasons: one, to avoid boredom, and two, to learn how to manage discomfort while running. Practicing fast running shows me I can run fast when I need to."

Mike Gallipeo, Huntington Beach, California: "I spent my first 4 years avoiding speedwork because I was afraid I would injure myself. For my last marathon, I added a day of speedwork a week, rotating tempo runs, hill repeats, and track work (800 repeats). My marathon time improved by 28 minutes! I am now a believer."

Rhondda Homfeldt, Ottawa, Illinois: "I didn't include speed training until my fourth marathon cycle. Now I do 1 day of speedwork a week, alternating between mile repeats, tempo runs, and hill repeats. It has helped me both physically and mentally. Marathon pace doesn't seem as hard anymore."

Eliza Drummond, Eugene, Oregon: "Speedwork provides spice to my training, breaking up the weekly mileage with some fun. I am fortunate enough to have a Thursday group where the coach provides the workouts. We just show up and do the work."

13

Defensive Strategies

You Cannot Set PRs If You Are Injured

I f you want to achieve success as a marathoner, you need to arrive at the starting line healthy. That's a given! You cannot finish the marathon if you fail to start. To do this, you need to avoid injuries. Defensive running strategies thus become an important part of your training plan. If you hope to have a long running career, determine what activities most often cause you to become injured, then avoid them. This is particularly true when it comes to overuse injuries that result from what might be called training errors.

Some physicians order injured runners to give up running. Several doctors offered me that advice earlier in my career—until I stopped going to doctors who were not runners themselves or who failed to understand the runner's mindset. For most of us, stopping running permanently is not an option. We want to run long distances. We want to run injury-free. Yet to run marathons is to court injury because of the high mileage involved in training for them. Jack H. Scaff, Jr., MD, founder of the Honolulu Marathon, says marathon running by definition is an "injury." Dr. Scaff is not advising people not to run marathons; he simply is stating what he considers to be a fact.

The late Michael L. Pollock, PhD, who directed the University of Florida Center for Exercise Science in Gainesville, identified intensity as the most common cause of running injuries. "People who only walk or jog short distances at slow paces don't become injured," he said.

Stan James, MD, the orthopedist from Eugene, Oregon, who performed arthroscopic surgery on Joan Benoit just three and a half months before her Olympic marathon victory, claims that most running injuries are the result of training errors. Avoid those errors, suggests Dr. James, and you can run injury free. Lyle J. Micheli, MD, founder of the Sports Medicine Division at Boston Children's Hospital and author of *The Healthy Runner's Handbook*, agrees: "Many of the injuries we see could have been prevented."

If you overtrain, something bad will happen.

Nevertheless, most successful training programs—including the ones presented in this book—are based on variations of the progressive overload theory. You gradually overload the system with more mileage or the same mileage at faster paces. To achieve peak performance, you train to just beneath the point where your body would break down if you crossed the line.

For most elite runners, the breaking point is somewhere beyond 100 miles per week, but not everyone is blessed with superior athletic ability. Podiatrists tell us their waiting rooms are filled with average runners who run 30 miles or more a week. Above that magic 30 miles seems to be where chondromalacia, plantar fasciitis, Achilles tendinitis, and other major injuries find us.

Logically, you just would not run beyond that 30 miles a week, but that hardly will suffice for marathoners. Surveys by *Runner's World* have suggested that when runners commit to running a marathon, they increase their weekly mileage over a period of time by 10 to 15 miles—from somewhere around 20 miles to between 30 and 40 miles a week. If podiatrists are correct, after reaching that level is when many of those runners call for appointments.

Megan Leahy, DPM, a Chicago podiatrist, comments: "Most of the injuries I encounter are runners who jumped into the sport too quickly, often with old or the wrong shoes." She suggests that many of her patients could have benefited from a gait analysis to make certain they had chosen the right shoes. Inserts or orthotics may relieve many problems; so can working with a physical therapist, but often that does not happen until after the injury.

If you are a marathoner seeking peak performance, the ideal is to determine—within a tenth of a mile, if possible—the weekly mileage at which your body self-destructs. Then you can train to the edge of disaster, occasionally pushing slightly over that edge to determine whether months and years of steady training (or a new pair of shoes) may have allowed you to nudge your breaking point to a new level, which will permit you to run a marathon or run that marathon faster.

Pushing to that edge must be done over a period of time. Elite runners spend many years gradually adapting their bodies to accept the stress of 100-mile weeks. They do not jump from 50 miles a week one month to 100 the next without getting hurt. First-time marathoners who try to increase their weekly mileage too rapidly, from fewer than 20 to more than 30, also are likely to get into trouble. They will develop injuries. Or they will become overtrained, resulting in diminished performance.

HOW OFTEN ARE RUNNERS INJURED?

Do runners get injured more often than other athletes? It sometimes seems so, because we often agonize over injuries so slight that we lose little or no training. I asked my online followers how often they got injured and got the following response.

How often did you get injured?	
I did not get injured	23%
Injured, I kept running	13%
Injured, I lost a few days	30%
Injured, I lost weeks	34%

This was, admittedly, an unscientific study, and I wondered how many uninjured runners did not bother to check a box. But the fact that a third of those responding reported injuries that kept them out of action for weeks troubled me. "I am the queen of injuries," reported Maggie Drake of Charlotte, North Carolina. "I had to take 7 months off because of an interior tibia stress fracture." This only proves that we all need to pay attention to the defensive strategies outlined in this chapter.

OVERTRAINING

Are you overtrained? Overtraining is not an injury per se. You are not hurt. Nothing is swollen; nothing is broken. You do not limp. It's just that when you run, your legs feel dead most of the time, both your workout and your race times start to deteriorate, and you enjoy running less and less. By overdoing it, you may be predisposing yourself to injury. If you overtrain, something bad will happen. Not *can* happen—will happen.

Marathon runners probably are more prone to overtraining than other runners simply because of the volume of training required. It stands to reason that if you train more, you increase your chances of becoming overtrained.

"A key contributor to the symptoms of overtraining is the loss of glycogen," states nutritionist Nancy Clark, RD, author of *Nancy Clark's Sports*

Nutrition Guidebook. Glycogen is the sugarlike substance that fuels your muscles and provides the readily available energy that permits them to contract efficiently. Glycogen debt can occur if you are not eating enough carbohydrates to match the amount you deplete during hard training sessions. "Your muscles need time to refuel," says Clark. "Rest days thus are an important part of any training program, but they often get overlooked by runners who underfuel and overtrain." Excessive training also seems to inhibit the body's conversion of fuel into energy. "Damaged muscles fail to store as much glycogen as fully functional muscles," adds Clark.

Some runners increase their training levels to reduce weight. They train for marathons to provide the means and incentive to slim down. But one common mistake is to combine an increase in mileage with a decrease in calorie consumption. Frequently, I get questions on the Internet from runners training for marathons who complain of energy loss, particularly at the end of their long runs. Inevitably, when I inquire, I discover that they were either dieting or following a low-carbohydrate regimen, which provides insufficient carbohydrates for high-mileage training. They became overtrained as much from their eating habits as from their training habits. One runner tweeted that he hoped to lose 10 to 15 pounds while training for a marathon and wondered whether a popular (low-carb) diet might help. I told him very emphatically, *no*, definitely not. Stick with a high-carb diet, and it also may help to consult with a nutritionist as to what that diet should be. We overlook the value of knowledgeable sports professionals at our own peril.

Your body is telling you to back off.

The overtrained runner may maintain speed but with poorer form and with greater expenditure of energy. David L. Costill, PhD, of the Human Performance Laboratory at Ball State University in Muncie, Indiana, cited one runner who, early in his training, could run a 6:00 mile pace at only 60 percent of his aerobic capacity. Later, when he became overtrained, the same runner had to use 80 percent of his capacity to maintain that pace. You may be able to train at your planned pace, but you will not train at it very long or go very far.

As athletes enlist all available muscle fibers in an attempt to maintain their training pace, they invariably exhaust their fast-twitch muscles before their slow-twitch muscles. This is one reason runners lose speed: Their fast-twitch muscles have become exhausted through intensive training.

But glycogen depletion is not the only problem. Another is microscopic damage to the muscle fibers, which tear, fray, and lose their resilience, like a rubber band that has been snapped too often. Despite analysis of blood and urine samples, researchers find it difficult to identify how or why chronically overtrained muscles lose their ability to contract.

KEEP A DIARY

The simplest defensive running strategy you can use is keeping a training diary. Determining where you made a mistake—that "training error" described by Dr. James—is the main reason for keeping a paper training diary, or a log if you record workouts on a computer. Learn the cause of that mistake and you are less likely to repeat it.

Your log can provide clues that you are overtraining. For example, if you have noted that you feel tired all the time, you may be training too hard. "Perceived exertion may give us our most important clues," says William P. Morgan, EdD, a sports psychologist at the University of Wisconsin at Madison. Here are some other symptoms to watch for.

Heavy legs. Your legs lose their snap—and speed. A run at an 8:00 pace feels like one at a 7:00 pace. Depleted muscle glycogen may be the cause. "You feel like you're running with glue on your shoes," says Dr. Costill.

Increased pulse rate. This is easily measured: Record your pulse each morning before you get out of bed, and cut back your training on days when it is higher than usual.

Sleep problems. You have trouble getting to sleep and may wake up several times during the night. Then you have to drag yourself out of bed in the morning. "Sleep dysfunctions often are a sign of overstress," says Dr. Costill.

Diminished sex drive. The romance has gone out of your life. Whether this lost interest in sex is related to lowered hormone levels caused by training or to just plain exhaustion, no one knows for sure.

Fear of training. You have trouble pushing yourself out the door to run each morning, so you sit and stretch longer. Your body is telling you to back off. "This is part of the psychological effect of overtraining," says Dr. Costill.

Sore muscles. Your muscles, particularly those of your legs, seem stiff. They may even be sore to the touch. The reason is muscle damage, caused by too much pounding on the roads. Some muscle soreness is natural after hard training sessions, but if it persists, that's a sign that you are working too hard.

I like to believe that individuals who use my training programs have a relatively low rate of injury. When people do get hurt, it is often for one of three reasons.

1. They started the program with insufficient base mileage.
2. They were first-time marathoners who followed the intermediate program rather than the novice program, because they had been running for several years and did not want to consider themselves "novices" or "joggers."
3. They ran their long runs at race pace or faster, believing it would get them in better shape to set a PR.

Each of these reasons could be branded by Dr. James as a training error.

AH-CHOO!

Another early warning sign of overtraining is the common cold, particularly right before an important race.

Upper-respiratory problems, from colds to the flu, are common among overtrained runners, claims Gregory W. Heath, DHSc, an exercise physiologist and epidemiologist at the Centers for Disease Control and Prevention in Atlanta. He notes that runners normally experience only half as many upper-respiratory infections as the general population. We are a healthy lot because of our lifestyles. Up to a certain point, exercise does boost immunity. But you lose this protection, claims Dr. Heath, if you race, and particularly if you race in marathons.

David C. Nieman, DrPH, director of the Human Performance Laboratory at Appalachian State University in Boone, North Carolina, surveyed participants in the Los Angeles Marathon and found that 40 percent had caught a cold during the 2 months prior to the race. By doing high-mileage training, runners lowered their resistance and became more susceptible to whatever cold bugs were floating around, even in the warm climate of Los Angeles.

Dr. Nieman discovered that if runners trained more than 60 miles a week, they doubled their risk of infection. He also found that in the week after the race, 13 percent of marathon finishers had caught colds, compared with 2 percent of runners who had not raced.

I believe in undertraining runners rather than overtraining them. The upper limit for my advanced marathon training programs falls somewhat below 60 weekly miles. I do not tell runners not to run more miles weekly; I simply believe they need to know what they are doing before they pursue a more aggressive program. Those who regularly run 60 miles a week and whose systems have adapted to that high load may not be at increased risk. Instead of being overtrained, they may be well trained. There is a fine line

It is a myth that you cannot get hurt crosstraining.

between being undertrained and overtrained; finding that line is not easy. It makes sense, nevertheless, to save your high-mileage training for months when the risk of infection is lower (spring through fall). Getting a flu shot at least once a year, usually in the fall, is important. You may not be able to avoid the flu entirely, but the shot will help ward off its worst symptoms, says Dr. Nieman.

Also, build a strong training base so that a week lost to a cold or flu won't be a serious setback. You should start your taper early enough to prevent problems during the week before the marathon. Finally, you need to be particularly wary following the race. "Spread of many viruses is hand to hand rather than airborne," says Dr. Heath, who recommends avoiding people with colds, washing your hands after contact, and, particularly, isolating yourself as much as possible before and after competition.

It is important to cut your training during a cold and cease it entirely if you have the flu (with an elevated temperature), because you may increase your chance of an injury while in a weakened condition. You can run a marathon with a cold without your symptoms greatly affecting performance (dehydration may be your worst problem), but running a marathon with the flu is definitely unwise. You might finish, but you could significantly compromise your immune system and incur health problems that can extend not merely weeks but months and even years, according to Dr. Nieman.

SLIDE INTO SPRING!

Start slow! I've said that several times already. One of the first lines of defense against injury is to quash your instinct to start training at full steam after a layoff. Many athletic injuries occur in the spring. After a sedentary winter, runners want to get out and start training at the same mileage level as in the fall. As a result, they get hurt.

As a high school coach, I discovered that young runners were particularly susceptible to injuries in both the spring and fall, a few weeks after track or cross-country season had begun. This was because they failed to train properly between seasons, and then they were forced to do too much too soon. The most common injury: shin splints, which was like an epidemic at the start of each season. Kids go from zero miles to high miles, and they get hurt.

It happens to adult runners, too, particularly those who have never run before but suddenly get inspired to take on a marathon. If inspiration comes a year before your marathon date, you probably have time to ease into a gentle training program that will take you from zero to 26 miles. If you have much less time available, you might want to pick as an interim goal a 5K, 10K, or half marathon and save your first marathon for later. Fortunately, more and more new runners seem to have discovered the half as an interim stop en route to a full.

Cross-training can lull even experienced runners into a false sense of security. Do not overvalue off-season training that does not involve running. During the period of my life when I remained in the Midwest all winter, I cross-country skied, and it got me into fabulous cardiovascular shape. But when the snow melted, I had to be cautious about bringing the same intensity to the running trails that I did to the ski trails.

I devised two strategies to help prevent this problem. First, instead of shifting completely from running to skiing as soon as snow covered the ground, I maintained a maintenance level of running—at least every other day. Frequently, I would jog a mile or so to the snow-covered golf course near my home with skis and poles in hand. And once the snow melted, I cut the intensity of my training during that transition period between winter and spring.

VARIETY

Nevertheless, cross-training can be an important means of preventing injury—if used wisely. One of the main causes of running injuries is the stress caused by the literally thousands of times your feet hit the ground when you run. If you have ever seen any slow-motion photography of what happens to the leg muscles during a single running stride, you would wonder how we survive even one lap around a track, much less a marathon. Swimming, skiing, cycling, and walking do not generate this ground impact.

When my wife, Rose, and I acquired a condo in Ponte Vedra Beach, Florida, we picked a location only a few minutes' walk from an ocean beach that provided a perfect running surface: flat and firm but also springy enough to minimize impact. Fortuitously, between condo and beach there was a fitness center with both a weight room and a swimming pool. After running on the beach, I could pump iron, then use the pool to both swim and run laps. Afterward, I could soak in the whirlpool to relieve sore muscles.

In the gym, I try to select exercises that simulate running as much as possible, but most cross-training fails to exercise the muscles specific to running. This is both good and bad, but in order to succeed as a runner, you need to train as a runner.

There is also the danger that you can cross-train yourself into an injury if you exercise excessively. Runners who cross-train on days between hard running bouts may do too much because they use different (read *unfatigued*) muscle groups. If you're not careful, you can convert an easy day into a hard day, and it will eventually catch up with you. It is a myth that you cannot get hurt cross-training.

If you can avoid gaps in your training caused by injuries, inevitably you will perform better as a runner.

We also are a nervous lot. One woman training for the marathon posted a message online, worried that she would lose fitness during the 3-week taper. She wondered if she could cross-train to compensate for the miles lost while tapering. My response was that if she was used to cross-training, she could continue with her other types of exercise; but it would be unwise to suddenly add new cross-training activities, particularly during the premarathon taper.

The whole purpose of the taper is to rest your muscles—all your muscles—by exercising significantly less. So, respect the taper! Cross-training the week after the marathon because you are too sore to run is also a very bad idea. I created an online postmarathon program primarily to discourage runners from resuming training too soon after their marathon efforts. The first 3 days after the marathon include no running and no cross-training, either.

Nevertheless, if you are prone to overuse injuries, substituting less stressful cross-training for some of your running may decrease your injuries and therefore your downtime. And if you can avoid gaps in your training caused by injuries, inevitably you will perform better as a runner.

MORE ON SPEEDWORK

Every running expert I know recommends speed training as the most effective means for improvement. (See the previous chapter.) But this can be dangerous advice if applied too zealously, particularly in training for a marathon.

A frequently asked question on social media comes from runners who have heard that speedwork can help them improve their marathon times. Should they start doing some fast running at the track? Not if they have just enrolled in a marathon program but have never before visited a track. Definitely not if the person asking the question is training for a first marathon. Even if that person has done speedwork in the past—such as someone with a track background—I say no. Only my advanced marathon programs include speedwork, but these programs are for experienced runners who are used to that type of training.

Speedwork is great—but only if properly planned.

It is not the speedwork itself that causes marathon runners to injure themselves in training but speedwork coupled with the progressively longer distances run during the marathon buildup. Early in my career, I learned that I could improve by increasing either the quality (speed) or the quantity (distance) of my workouts, but I could not do both at the same time without risking injury. Marathoners should include speedwork in their training programs only after an initial buildup to high mileage and a subsequent cutback.

TAKE THE TRAIL

Here's another training option for runners wanting to avoid injury: trail running. I believe in trail running, partly because I love to run through the woods, but also because there is less chance of getting injured on soft but firm surfaces. Yet I have noticed that runners unused to varying trail surfaces are prone to injury when they run cross-country. This was borne out by my cross-country team at the beginning of the fall season, as well as the track team when it trained on trails after the long winter hiatus. The less dedicated runners, who had failed to work out during the off-season, tripped over roots or twisted their ankles while stepping in holes, but this never seemed to happen to runners who trained on trails year-round.

One exception: Liz, the fastest girl on the team my first two years coaching at Elston High School in Michigan City. Liz trained hard year-round, but she had a very low and efficient stride. While running, she barely cleared the ground, skimming along maybe an inch above the surface. Biomechanical scientists will tell you that this is a very efficient way to run. You waste energy if you have too high a stride. Unfortunately, it seemed that Liz fell victim to every hidden root on the trails we ran at the Indiana Dunes State Park near Chesterton, Indiana. But Liz was good at picking herself up and, being young, she experienced the occasional bruise but not any serious injuries.

Nevertheless, if you are going to race on roads, you need to train on roads to accustom your muscles to the impact. When preparing for a marathon, I usually do a much higher percentage of my running on the roads than when I'm training for shorter events, such as track and cross-country races.

With the increase in the number of fitness centers and with the number of treadmills at those centers, many runners have begun to train indoors on such devices, particularly when winter winds blow. Or in the summer, as an air-conditioned option when it gets too hot. Christine Clark of Alaska won the 2000 Olympic marathon trials despite having done most of her training on a treadmill. But she ran outdoors as well.

Making the switch from treadmill to pavement in spring sometimes can be tricky. There exists a subtle but important difference between running on a moving belt, which can carry you along, and running on pavement, where all of the propulsion is yours. Runners who trust the numbers related to pace on their treadmills are sometimes surprised to find that they have to work harder to maintain that pace outdoors. Or sometimes easier if the treadmill is improperly calibrated to balance indoor miles with outdoor miles. Nevertheless, treadmills are a blessing for many runners, generally providing a more cushioned running surface than the roads. Treadmill running can help prevent impact injuries. But if you set the treadmill incline too high, so that you are running more on your toes, you can develop other injuries, particularly plantar fasciitis and Achilles tendinitis.

BUY BETTER SHOES

One way to diminish road shock is to wear properly cushioned shoes. Running shoe companies spend millions of dollars on research and technology to design shoes that help prevent injuries. Various energy-absorbing materials, along with air built into or pumped into your shoes, can decrease the impact of running on either asphalt or concrete.

One possible reason that men's marathon times have improved by nearly 20 minutes in the last half century may be better footwear and, as a result, fewer training injuries. A word of caution, however: Shoes that are too spongy (so soft that they offer little support) may destabilize the foot and contribute to injury.

Choose your footwear very carefully. For example, heavier runners need shoes that offer more support than those designed for lighter runners. You may also need more than one type of shoe. I have a built-in rack in my basement on which I stack my various athletic shoes, each pair for a specific purpose.

I wear heavy, protective shoes on easy days when I run slow. When I run fast, I prefer a light shoe, and I often wear racing flats for my speed workouts and a semilight pair for long runs. When I run smooth trails, I wear a flexible, light shoe; uneven trails may require shoes with studs on the bottom. At the track, I may don spikes for repeats. I also have cycling shoes and ski boots and water socks for the beach. Finally, I sometimes run through snow in mukluks similar to those worn by polar explorers.

The secret of endurance is to stay uninjured.

Every shoe has its own place in a runner's shoe inventory, and certain shoes that work well in one setting may not perform well in another. Runners who wear inflexible road shoes in the woods may increase their chance of injury on the uneven ground. Cross-training shoes may be suitable for weekend warriors who exercise infrequently, but I am not convinced they belong in the inventory of any serious endurance athlete.

Listing makes and models of running shoes doesn't do much good in a book such as this. Even shoe surveys by *Runner's World* frequently lose relevance as shoe companies continue to change and update their styles (not always improving them). The best source of information on running shoes is—surprise, surprise—specialty running shoe stores, which often employ salespeople who are runners like us. Some stores use treadmills so the salespeople can observe the customers running in the shoes.

Or they will watch you run on the sidewalk out front—as long as you don't go too far!

Although I have been sponsored at various points in my career by different shoe companies, I sometimes run shoeless, at least during warm weather. I did this long before the barefoot fad created by the bestselling book *Born to Run*. When I run on grass or sand or sometimes in deep water, I go barefoot because I believe that it stretches and strengthens the muscles in my feet. At least a few innovative coaches prescribe a certain amount of barefoot running (a few miles a week) for their athletes. I have even raced without shoes, running 5000 meters barefoot on London's Crystal Palace track in 1972, setting a masters record that lasted a quarter century. Telling you that I run barefoot will not endear me to the shoe companies, but it is all part of my defensive running approach.

STRETCH AND STRENGTHEN

Learning how to stretch is another way to minimize injury. Add to that strength training. As to the former, the best time to stretch a muscle is after it is warmed up. Track runners typically jog a mile or two, then stretch or do calisthenic exercises before beginning the intense part of a workout.

Long-distance runners are less likely to pause in the middle of a long run to stretch, although maybe we should do so more often. I will stretch before long runs and in the middle of intense workouts, but my preferred time to stretch is after the workout. Every runner should adopt a stretching regimen that is convenient and comfortable.

Strength training is important for both conditioning and injury prevention. I lift weights and/or use exercise machines regularly, but it is wise to cut back on your strength training during the marathon mileage buildup. Light weights and high repetitions seem to work best for marathoners. Do not—repeat, do not—overdo strength training if you want success as a marathoner. I recommend less or no lifting the last 3 to 6 weeks before the race at the time when you are peaking near 20 miles. You may be able to continue lifting safely, but why take a chance? If a specific injury threatens, I am quick to seek advice related to my strength-training routine from a trainer or physical therapist. Some exercises will speed your recovery; others may slow it.

Part of my long-term success as a runner has come from avoiding the types of injuries that require extensive rehabilitation. During more than a half century of running, I have had very little downtime: a sore Achilles tendon now and then, a strained knee once, plantar fasciitis on another occasion. Nothing much. No surgery. And hey, my main event as a track-and-field athlete was the 3000-meter steeplechase, a race of nearly 2 miles that required me to hurdle four 3-foot barriers per lap plus a fifth barrier with a 12-foot water jump behind it. The 'chase, as we called it, was most definitely a contact event, particularly if you added in other runners elbowing for position. I am either smart or lucky or I have what Dr. Costill describes as a "bulletproof body," one that is biomechanically sound (or maybe it is a combination of all three). Although two of these factors are out of your control, you can be smart about your training by including stretching and strengthening as part of your routine.

DON'T GET HURT TWICE

If you experience a specific injury the first time, I'll allow you to alibi that injury away as an "accident." If you are hurt a second time, you have what tennis fans call an *unforced error*. You need to change, do something different, to prevent injury repeats. After experiencing an injury serious enough that standard remedies such as ice, anti-inflammatories, and rest fail to provide relief, a runner needs not only to seek medical advice but also to consult his or her training diary to identify the training patterns that contributed to the injury. Coming off an injury or a period of reduced training mileage, runners also often reinjure themselves, says Russell H. Pate, PhD, chairman of the department of exercise science at the University of South Carolina in Columbia. "Runners think, 'I can do 40 miles a week again,' but their bodies aren't ready," he says.

After following the daily training of 600 runners for a year, Dr. Pate identified two major predictors for injuries: a previous injury and heavy training. "If you got injured once and don't modify your training, you probably will get injured again," he says.

For runners doing heavy training, three factors determined whether they would be reinjured: frequency, mileage, and whether they ran marathons. A critical problem was the runners' approach to training. "Too rapid a buildup is a critical factor in injuries," says Dr. Pate. "You need to know your limitations." Once you determine that, you can modify your training to prevent future injury.

MOST COMMON RUNNING INJURIES

What are the most common running injuries? While writing another book, *Masters Running*, I surveyed more than five hundred athletes over age 40 to find out which injuries plagued them the most. Here are the results of that survey. Respondents were allowed to check more than one injury, which explains why the frequency numbers add up to more than 100 percent.

Injury	Frequency
Muscle pull	32%
Knee injury	30%
Plantar fasciitis	26%
Nonrunning injury	22%
Iliotibial band injury	20%
Achilles tendinitis	17%
Shin splits	16%
Stress fracture	9%
Health-related problems	8%
No injuries	10%

If you can determine which injury plagues you the most, you can figure out the best defensive strategies to avoid it. A running log—computer or paper—is often the best ally for figuring out what went wrong.

One additional strategy I use in preventing injury is to obtain therapeutic massages. I use the services of two massage therapists: one in Indiana and one in Florida. Typically, I schedule a massage once every 2 weeks, more frequently if I am training hard for a specific race. And I will often schedule a massage for a day or two before or after the race, particularly if it is a marathon. I also have found that a massage is the perfect antidote to jet lag, although it sometimes requires skill to locate a massage therapist in a different city or country. While the free (or low-cost) postrace massages available at marathons feel good, it is better to get a massage 24 to 48 hours after the race, while your muscles are recovering. Professional athletes often get more frequent massages. If I were a pro whose income depended on my performance, I would get massages more often than I do now.

Therapists sometimes suggest that massage can soothe and heal fatigued muscles, but research on the subject is scanty. I do not need a scientist to tell me whether a massage works or not. I am convinced that the most important benefit from massage is the relaxation effect. A relaxed muscle is less likely to get injured.

But you should also learn how to rest. My novice programs include rest on 2 days of the week: Monday and Friday. My intermediate and advanced programs nibble away at those days of rest, but consider that for many advanced runners, an easy run of 3 miles could be considered rest. Unfortunately, sometimes injuries force unwanted rest days upon us, at which point we need to shout, "Help," and make an appointment with a sports medicine specialist. This happens often at the last minute, before an important race for which we have trained hard, often too hard.

Podiatrist Megan Leahy, DPM, tells me: "In my practice, I often see overuse injuries from the BQ athlete who pushed through just a tad too much and sought treatment a tad too late. It's challenging to come up with a treatment plan for these runners. My runner's heart wants to do everything I can to get them to the finish line, but oftentimes I have to put on my doctor's hat and give more conservative, safe and healthy advice." As runners, it is important to look at our miles as a lifetime journey. A break here and there can be difficult, but knowing when to program rest can ultimately contribute to the longevity of a healthy lifestyle.

GETTING OLDER

Longevity is something, as runners, we all should seek. Basic training principles apply to all runners, but the specifics may vary greatly. Although running offers a marvelous means of diminishing the effects of aging, the body eventually begins to slow, and, as you get older, certain cautions are in order.

Instead of 1 day's rest after a hard speed session or a long run, you may need 2 days or more. And standard training programs may not work for you if they predispose you to injury. Regardless of what it says in this and other books about improvement, at a certain age you may need to eliminate some of the workouts that make you more vulnerable to getting hurt. This could include interval running on a track, hill training, fartlek, and other workouts that involve stop/start activities. *Be consistent!* This is what older runners learn because the secret of endurance is to stay uninjured. All you need to do is run steadily every week, and, whether or not you improve, you will at least maintain your ability as best you can.

Dynamic repair is a fancy title for rest coined by Bob Glover, a supervisor of coaches for the New York Road Runners. Glover considers rest to be a commonly overlooked component of any successful training program, and he believes that less training is sometimes best. "When in doubt, the coach should suggest less, and I've gotten softer and softer every year," he says. "By minimizing injury and getting a person to improve gradually instead of rapidly, you'll have the most success. The old coach's mentality was to get out there and crack the whip: survival of the fittest. But how many people ended up on the junk heap along the way?"

Inevitably, if you can avoid injury, you can run long distances for the longest time. Defensive running may be the best training strategy.

14

Water Therapy

If Injured, Take to the Pool

As a high school runner leading into her freshman track season, Megan Leahy experienced a stress fracture leaping off boxes during plyometric drills. Earlier in the year, I had coached Megan in cross-country. Her arrival was like that of a lightning bolt, as she immediately claimed the role as number one on the team. Though fast, she also was a fragile runner, one just beginning to develop the skills that would allow her to succeed in future races.

After Megan's injury I conferred with her track coach but also her mother, Joanne, herself a talented marathon runner. We decided to throw Megan into the pool.

Not for punishment, but to speed her recovery. For the remainder of the spring, while her teammates had fun running in track meets, Megan, under her mom's strict supervision, ground it out day after day, clad in a flotation vest, mimicking running motions in deep water, maintaining fitness while avoiding impact.

Alas, by the time the doctor cleared Megan to run again, the season had ended. Nevertheless, she would benefit from what at first seemed like wasted training. Injured again at the start of her senior year in cross-country, Megan returned to the pool. She started running again barely in time for the countdown to State. A second-place finish earned her a scholarship to Indiana University. (Megan's team also won State, its second title in two years, although under the guidance of another coach.)

As a marathoner, you may or may not be tempted to run cross-country trails or 1500 meters on the track, but you can profit from what Megan Leahy learned while pool running.

As Megan discovered, pool running does work. In fact, I submit that pool running—specifically using a flotation device to run in the deep end of a pool—is *the* very best form of cross-training if you are recovering from injury and unable to run. Pool running cannot substitute entirely for running on roads, but it comes closer to mimicking running than any other cross-training activity. In an article published by *Runner's World*, Cindy Kuzma quotes bio-mechanist John Mercer: "Deep-water running isn't a new idea. Runners borrowed it decades ago from horse trainers who used it to rehab or supplement their animals' mileage."

Pool running is the best form of cross-training.

Citing scientific studies, Mercer suggests that deep-water training not only allows runners to maintain cardiovascular fitness, but also to improve it. Three reasons exist for why runners should embrace pool running.

1. **Recovering from injury:** Running in a flotation vest comes closest to mimicking real running on land. Cycling or using various gym-based machines allows you to maintain cardiovascular fitness but fails to mimic the running movement. Mercer suggests that the blood-pumping pressure of water actually may speed healing.

2. **Avoiding injury:** Runners who flirt with injury by running too often or too fast can cross-train in a pool to add variety to their training. Jennifer Conroyd, founder of the firm Fluid Running,

which offers flotation vests for runners under the brand name H2Go, recommends one or two pool workouts a week as the best mix with running.

3. **Maintaining fitness:** Forget performance. Forget injury prevention. One of the best reasons to convert to pool running is to stay in shape. According to *Aerobics* author Kenneth H. Cooper, MD, physical exercise, almost any kind of exercise, has been shown to extend life-span six to nine more years but also to improve the quality of that life.

That has been my goal. My wife and I spend half our year in Indiana, half in Florida. In Indiana, I live across the street from Lake Michigan with its soft, sandy bottom. A regular workout routine is to run chest-deep in water parallel to shore. In Florida, we belong to a club featuring a heated outdoor pool with lanes marked for swimmers. No deep water, unfortunately, so after a workout in the gym, I swim several laps, then run several more. In all honesty, I swim as much for relaxation as for fitness.

Consider the three types of training you can do in a pool:

1. **Deep-water running:** This is the best form of cross-training both for healing injuries and for preventing injuries. If my Florida pool had a deep end, I definitely would add deep-water running to my workout routine.
2. **Swimming:** This is a sport that strengthens muscles not used by runners. Although too much upper-body muscle can slow runners down, the fact that swimming ignores running muscles offers a huge advantage for injury recovery and prevention.
3. **Shallow-water running:** Shallow in this case would be anywhere from waist- to chest-deep. Lower impact than running on the roads makes this a great option, particularly to prevent injuries rather than to cure an injury. I love running in chest-deep water, one reason being you can swivel your head and see what's happening around you. My wife, Rose, participates in a water

aerobics class in the area of the pool next to the lap-swimming lanes, so I get to listen to all their gossip.

Megan Leahy describes what she learned as a pool runner: "I definitely felt pool running was far more forgiving than running outdoors. For example, I would never dream of doing speedwork on the track on back-to-back days, but I definitely had no problem doing speedwork daily in the pool."

This was necessary, Megan felt, because she found it more difficult to get her heart rate up in the pool. (This is generally true among competitive swimmers versus competitive runners.) To compensate, Megan would remove the flotation belt and tread water in the deep end. "My form definitely was sacrificed, but I was able to get my heart rate up easier."

At Indiana University after graduation from high school, Megan continued to pool run, though less in the deep end with a flotation belt, because the diving team occupied that area. "I was afraid of divers landing on my head," she says.

After ending her collegiate career, Megan decided to become a podiatrist. Megan Leahy, DPM, now practices in Chicago. "I suffered every injury imaginable in school," she admits," so I picked a profession where I could help others avoid the same."

Consider blending pool running with your regular running and cross-training, and you may never need to visit Dr. Leahy's office.

TRAINING IN THE WATER

Marathoners recovering from an injury can use various pool-based exercises for their recovery. Depending on the severity of your injury, you may need anywhere from 1 to 8 or more weeks to recover. Do so by substituting pool-based exercises for whatever running workouts you might have been doing at the time of your injury. At the end of 4 weeks—assuming you have begun to recover—begin to blend regular running (indoors or outdoors) with your training in a pool. Hopefully after 8 weeks of pool running, you will be ready to resume running full time. If not, continue in the pool until recovered. Use the following chart as a *pattern* for your pool running; be willing to substitute or innovate depending on the facilities available to you.

Pool Running

DEFINITION OF TERMS

Deep = Deep-water running with flotation vest

Swim = Swimming in lap pool or lake

Run/Swim = Run and/or swim in shallow pool

Run = Run indoors or out (or stationary bike)

Week	Mon	Tue	Wed	Thu	Fri	Sat	Sun
1	Rest	Deep 15 min	Swim 20 min	Deep 15 min	Rest	Run/ Swim 30 min	Deep 30 min
2	Rest	Swim 25 min	Deep 20 min	Swim 25 min	Rest	Run/ Swim 30 min	Deep 40 min
3	Rest	Deep 25 min	Swim 30 min	Deep 25 min	Rest	Run/ Swim 30 min	Deep 50 min
4	Rest	Swim 25 min	Deep 20 min	Swim 25 min	Rest	Run/ Swim 30 min	Deep 60 min
5	Rest	Run 15 min	Swim 30 min	Run 15 min	Rest	Run/ Swim 30 min	Deep 60 min
6	Rest	Run 20 min	Deep 30 min	Run 20 min	Rest	Run/ Swim 30 min	Run 30 min
7	Rest	Run 15 min	Run/ Swim 30 min	Run 15 min	Rest	Run 15 min	Run 45 min
8	Rest	Run 30 min	Run/ Swim 30 min	Run 30 min	Rest	Run 30 min	Run 60 min

15

Planning for Peak Performance

Think Far Ahead

Aiming at key races is the best way to achieve peak performance in long-distance events. This is where progressive training directed toward a certain event comes in: You start from a low point of conditioning and build to a high point. You compete in a race or a series of races: a 10K, a half marathon, a marathon.

You then relax your training and begin to contemplate your next goal. And maybe in between, you do some speedwork aimed at improving your basic speed before going back to an endurance-based program.

This is what coaches call *periodization*. The late New Zealand coach Arthur Lydiard probably deserves most of the credit for popularizing this approach following the success of his gold medal Olympians Murray Halberg and Peter Snell. At different periods of the year, you use different training approaches, sometimes setting interim goals while still focused on your ultimate goal. For most readers of this book (given its title), that ultimate goal would be either finishing, or running fast, in a marathon.

More than any other event, the marathon lends itself to this approach. Although some runners run a dozen or more half marathons or marathons a year, most distance runners are content to run one or two during any given 12-month period. Many runners will run a single marathon in a lifetime. Usually these races are selected well in advance, allowing ample time for a buildup to peak performance.

How do you plan for peak performance? How do you adjust your training schedule in anticipation of a specific race? How do you guarantee that you can follow that planned schedule and maximize your chances for success—and enjoyment? Unfortunately, there exists no magic formula, no magic mileage, no magic mold into which you can put runners.

Nevertheless, certain guidelines can help you achieve peak performance.

YOU NEED TIME

If you expect to peak for a specific race—whether a mile or a marathon—you need time. You need time to plan, time to establish a base, time to progress, and time to taper properly.

How much time? For a short-distance event on the track or an important 5K or half marathon on the roads, you probably need at least 2 to 3 months of preparation. If you are talking marathon, 4 to 5 months is probably enough time for most first-timers. (My marathon training programs last 18 weeks but assume you arrive at the starting point with some level of fitness.) For experienced runners seeking improvement, 6 months is probably minimal, and 12 would be better. Former world-class marathoner Benji Durden of Boulder, Colorado, designed an 84-week schedule for me to use in my book *How to Train*. It involved a preliminary buildup to one test marathon, then a peak buildup to a second PR effort, with half marathons serving as interim goals. Those with Olympic aspirations must think four years ahead. But even if your goals are less than Olympian, you may need

> **To achieve success, you need to plan for success.**

to do the same. Is this marathon a onetime event to fulfill a bucket list, or will running long-distance races become part of a major lifestyle change? If you are a first-time marathoner, you may not even know the answer to that question yet, but to achieve success, you need to plan for success. You want enough time to execute a well-organized plan that will bring you to the starting line in the best shape of your life. If you do not do that, you are not peaking. And you have not learned to apply the principles of periodization.

PERIODIZATION

Periodization is a term used by coaches to describe a system of training that extends over a period of weeks, months, and even years. Although New Zealand coach Arthur Lydiard did not invent the term, he certainly pioneered the division of a runner's training into different periods of time leading to a specific goal. For at least some of Arthur's runners (such as Murray Halberg and Peter Snell), that goal was winning an Olympic gold medal.

Here is how periodization might work for runners coming off one marathon who want to prepare for another. Some periods may blend with others.

Rest: After a marathon, you need an extended period of active rest for 3 to 6 weeks before beginning to train hard again.

Endurance-I: Miles, and lots of them, are the key to success in long-distance running. Lydiard even had half-milers such as Snell running 23-milers for their base training. Most endurance-trained marathoners may be able to skip this period—or postpone it until later.

Strength: To run fast, you need strong muscles. Lydiard's athletes ran hills. Interval training on the track also can improve strength and speed. To run fast, however, you need to cut back on mileage during this period.

(continued)

> *Speed:* Marathoners can improve their speed by racing at shorter distances—specifically, 5K and 10K. The best time to do this is during a period when you are not increasing mileage. The speed and strength periods may overlap.
>
> *Endurance-II:* This is the final mileage buildup leading to the marathon itself. My 18-week training programs allow runners to increase their longest runs from 6 to 20 miles.
>
> *Taper:* Do not overlook this important period. You cannot achieve peak performance unless you are well rested.
>
> *The marathon:* Run your fastest, then periodize your training again for your next major effort.

PICKING A GOAL

Before you make a plan, you need a goal. If you want to float along from week to week, training the way you feel, racing whenever you want to, that's fine. Running need not always be the relentless pursuit of one big event after another. We all need downtime to renew ourselves psychologically, to gather ourselves for the next push. Sometimes I take a year or more off from serious training and racing. Bill Bowerman was the late—and great—track coach at the University of Oregon. Bill also was one of the founders of Nike. I have written often about the Bowerman approach, which features hard days and easy days. But taking Bill's approach to an extreme, I often plan hard years and easy years. Sometimes not having a goal for any one year may even fit into a career approach to marathoning.

Usually I set goals at the beginning of each year. Sometimes my goals are a set of times I want to improve at various distances—or maybe there are a number of races I want to do well in. For much of my career, I chose to peak for the World Masters Championships, a track-and-field meet, which takes place at two-year intervals. This strategy allowed me to win four gold medals, nine medals overall (including silver and bronze). Other times, I would peak for a marathon.

Marathons do lend themselves to goal setting because of the extra effort required both to train for them and to compete well in them—and simply because of the magic of the marathon itself. But setting a goal involves not merely selecting an event or events but also deciding what you expect from your participation in that event. Is your goal just to finish? Is your goal a PR? Is your goal victory—or at least placing high in your age group? Or maybe you are just out to have a good time. You need to determine your principal goal first, and only after that can you begin to make plans.

> **It is possible to have subgoals, or a series of goals.**

It is also possible to have subgoals, or a series of goals. You may want to run some preliminary races—and run them well—as interim contests before the main race that interests you most. First-time marathoners probably need a few races under their belts at distances from 5K to the half marathon, if only so they can get some hint as to what their marathon finishing time might be. Sometimes I select a primary goal (such as running a fast marathon), expecting to use it as a stepping-stone to a greater goal (running a faster marathon).

On the other hand, if your goals are too many or too diverse, you may have difficulty achieving your main goal.

GAME PLAN

Once you set your goal, you can make a plan to achieve it. Here is where training logs and diaries come in handy, particularly for those of us who have been running for more than a few years. Whether or not I actually pull individual diaries down from the shelf, I will at least mentally review what has worked for me in the past and what has not. Even if I decide to take a totally different approach—say, low-mileage training instead of high-mileage—it will be pursued after considerable reflection.

I used to do a lot of my preliminary planning on airplanes as I returned from major events. If, as so often happened, I was on an overseas flight, I would have plenty of time trapped in a tight seat with nothing better to do than think. Invariably the food was terrible, and I already had seen what probably was a bland movie, so what better time for considering future goals? Sometimes I would pull out a notebook and jot down dates and times or tap away at my laptop.

Inevitably, however, I fine-tune any plans after returning home. Even though my life revolves around cyberspace, I still feel most comfortable using paper and pen for planning. On a large sheet, I draw a homemade calendar with large blocks for each date. I list major events in appropriate boxes, usually drawing a red border around the important box, the day on which I want to hit my peak. I may list certain workouts I want to run or distances (daily or weekly) I want to achieve. Or I may use the calendar to record how my training is going. I record the distance of my long runs and my weekly miles, and I may plot key speed workouts in advance or record them after they occur. I do the same with races and my times at those races. This is in addition to my regular log, where I record more specific details about individual workouts every day.

Keeping a training diary is like writing love letters to yourself.

Is this a little *too* organized? Maybe, but planning of just that sort has been a major factor in my success as a runner.

"Why train if you don't have a goal?" asks Paula Sue Russell of Findlay, Ohio.

Rhondda Homfeldt from Ottawa, Illinois, says: "Big races and hotels around them fill fast now. If you don't plan your next-year goals, you'll be running small races instead of big ones or sleeping in a tent."

"Planning is essential for me in order to avoid the postmarathon blues," says Amber Balbier of Dallas, Texas. "I tend to feel sad as early as the taper, so planning the next goal helps drive those blues away."

Reinhold Messner, one of the great mountain climbers of all time, once said: "Each goal achieved is equally a dream destroyed." Runners need to keep resetting goals as well as reinventing themselves.

THE DIARY APPROACH

Despite having three decades' worth of diaries on a shelf in my office, I now record workouts on a computer. Many runners go to my website and print or download one of the training programs for novice, intermediate, or advanced runners. Or they sign up for one of my interactive programs, where I send them daily email messages telling them what to run. Runners using my interactive programs find it quite easy to modify dates and numbers to fit specific marathon training needs, then afterward record each workout with a few numbers or in infinite detail. In many respects, keeping a training diary is like writing love letters to yourself.

Planning is where time and goal come together. If you have a specific period of time in which to achieve a specific goal, you can plan accordingly—to a point, of course. You cannot predict whether the wind will be in your face or the weather will be too warm. But you can plan almost every other aspect of your marathon training so you will reach the starting line ready to perform to the best of your ability.

"Figure out the key sessions you need for your program," Dr. Russell H. Pate once told me. "Get them in there, then surround them with those kinds of recovery activities that allow you to continue over a period of time. Build your program on priorities. The highest priority is attached to the key, hard sessions."

Comparing Dr. Pate's recommendation with my Novice 1 marathon training program, the key workout is the weekly long run. Second in importance is the midweek "sorta-long" run. Looking at my toughest training program, Advanced 2, in addition to back-to-back runs on weekends, the two speed workouts on Tuesdays and Thursdays are important for runners at that level.

Dr. Pate summarizes: "The secret to success in long-distance running is not what type of workouts you do, whether high or low intensity, but how those workouts are structured into a specific program and incorporated throughout a training year—and for the length of a career as well."

TIME OUT

How important is rest? If you've been reading carefully, you should understand by now just how important it is.

While you are choosing your goal and planning your approach, you may want to take time to relax: a planned vacation, not necessarily away from running, but away from training at maximum effort. *Rest* is a word you have encountered before in this book, and it is a word you will encounter again.

Rest is not always entirely optional, of course. If you have completed a marathon, you may be forced into a period of recuperation that could last a week, a month, or more. This time is necessary not only to allow sore muscles to recover but also to permit rejuvenation of the spirit.

It may take more time for the spirit to recover than the muscles. Psychiatrists write about postmarathon depression. At a premarathon lecture in Chicago, Joan Benoit Samuelson referred to it as PMS. At first many of the women in the audience thought she was talking about premenstrual syndrome. When Joanie explained she meant postmarathon syndrome, women as well as men gave a nervous laugh.

At least in the aftermath of a marathon, there usually is a period of well-deserved euphoria because of a peak performance, particularly one that involved so much preparation. First-time marathoners are more susceptible than others because they have passed—for better or worse—

through a unique experience. They wonder, "What do I do next?" and often there is no immediate answer.

One year, Ron Gunn of Southwestern Michigan College and I took a large number of runners from his beginning running class to the Honolulu Marathon. The morning after the race, we planned a short walk along the beach from our hotel to the Royal Hawaiian Hotel for brunch. Nearly everybody appeared wearing the finisher shirt they had won the previous day. Inevitably, of course, that revered shirt gets thrown into the dirty laundry. Regardless of whether you immediately select your next goal, take ample time to enjoy the just-completed experience before setting your next goal.

A few more miles this week.

BEGIN WITH BASE

In many respects, the base period (when you run easy without worrying about pace or distance) is an extension of the rest period. Usually within a week after finishing a marathon, muscle soreness will have almost completely disappeared, and you can begin to run comfortably again. But you need time to stabilize your training. Do not rush immediately into all-out training for your next goal. If you do, you are liable to crash some weeks or months later.

Runners tend to have a comfortable base level of training, a weekly maintenance mileage that they can accomplish almost effortlessly. For many veteran runners, that base level is about 15 or 20 miles. They do not need to aim at running that much; it just happens. Most of us enjoy exercise. So we head out the door 3 or 4 or 5 days a week without thinking about where we are going or how far or how fast. A runner might end the week with 15 to 20 miles recorded in his or her training log and not think much about the numbers. That is the base maintenance level to which we as runners periodically return. We run enough to maintain a reasonable amount of fitness. It is like setting the number on your thermostat down from 70 to 65 degrees before going to bed.

Then, when we have a specific race we want to run—a half marathon, a marathon—we push the button that resets our thermostats to a slightly higher level, enough to allow us to reach our next goal. We have an edge on first-time marathoners because we know the routine, but we still train in the same manner, moving from a somewhat low level to a somewhat higher level of fitness.

Practically every beginner's program depends on gradually increasing distance, usually on a weekly basis. A few more miles this week; a few more miles than that the next week. Nobody has been able to come up with a better approach to building fitness, and I doubt anybody ever will. It is the old story of Milo (the ancient Greek wrestler) and the bull. You start lifting a calf when it is young, and by the time the calf grows into a heavy bull, you have the strength to throw people out of the ring in the Olympics.

The same is true with running: You take people running 15 to 25 miles a week, and by adding a few miles a week over a period of 18 weeks, you get them up near 40 to 50 miles weekly. You take people capable of running an hour (or half a dozen miles) continuously and help them progress to where they can run for 3 to 4 hours or more (or about 20 miles).

Fatigue, diet, and sleep can affect the intensity of your training.

If you are talking peak performance, however, you need to do more than spend 4 months adding a mile a week and increasing your final long workout to 20 miles. You need to take sufficient time (or have a sufficient base) to arrive at that level probably at least 2 months before the marathon—and hold at that level.

Excuse me, first-timers, if I take some time to preach to the choir. For experienced runners, a single 20-miler is not enough. For peak performance, you need to develop the ability to run 20-milers repeatedly (two or three times) without undue fatigue and without overtraining.

Some runners go beyond marathon distance in their training. At one point I progressed to 31-mile (50K) workouts, but I eventually decided that it was counterproductive, at least for me. Running that far took too much time, and I had to slow down too much to achieve that distance. Recovery took longer.

I figured there must be a better means of adding mileage. My solution was to add a second, shorter long run to my training week, usually about two-thirds of the distance of the longest run: 10 miles if my long run was 15; 13 to 15 miles if my long run was 20. It is possible to increase your long and sorta-long runs simultaneously, but a more sensible approach is to stabilize your long run near 20 miles, then begin a progression featuring a second workout.

Every third or fourth week, depending on how I felt, I would take an extra day or two of rest. I would back down from my weekly mileage and maybe skip my long run that week. That allowed me to gather strength so that I could progress to a still-higher level.

ADD INTENSITY

Another standard approach for elite runners is to increase the intensity of their training sessions. One way to increase overall intensity is to do your runs at various distances faster. When I peak for spring marathons, this happens naturally. As the weather warms, I can run more fluidly in shorts and a T-shirt than I can in the multilayered outfit I wear in colder weather. Similarly, before fall marathons, I find I can run more comfortably (and faster) as the weather cools, at least to a point. Some natural speeding is acceptable as you increase distance and improve fitness, but to push too fast, too far, too soon raises the specter of overtraining and injury.

It is usually a good idea to run your distance workouts at a comfortable pace and increase intensity in separate speed sessions. In fact, most experienced runners may decrease their mileage at least slightly when moving from the distance phases to the speed phases of their peak training plans. Various forms of speedwork, particularly interval training, lend themselves to progressive training of this sort.

A typical speed progression would be to start with running 10 × 400 in 90 seconds with a 400 jog in between, then over 10 successive weeks lower the time 1 second a week until you are capable of running 10 × 400 in 80 seconds. Another approach would be to begin at 5 × 400 and add an extra repetition at the same pace each week until you achieve 10 × 400 or more.

Do not let the numbers frighten you. Progressions such as those just described work only if you begin conservatively and do not pick an end goal beyond your capabilities. Many runners (including me now) would find it difficult to run a single 400 in 90 seconds, much less use that as their starting point. No matter. We all play with the hands we are dealt and succeed or fail at various levels, depending on our abilities.

Hill training is another means of increasing workout intensity. You can run sprints up hills as a form of speed training or shift to hilly courses for your long runs. Preparing for the Chicago Marathon, which has a relatively flat course, I would select flat courses for my long runs. When I prepared for a hillier marathon, such as Boston, I trained over hillier courses, at least during the closing stages of my training. I also included some downhill repeats, since Boston is a point-to-point course that drops in elevation. This can make for very fast times, but you need to be prepared for the pounding your legs (especially your quadriceps) will take on the downhill portion of the race.

One runner complained to me online that in the closing stages of her marathon, she experienced calf cramps that slowed her down, enough to prevent her from achieving a time that would qualify her for Boston. Probing, I discovered that in order to get that BQ, she had chosen a point-to-point downhill course with an 800-foot drop in it. Fair enough, but then she had failed to add the downhill training that would help her achieve her goal.

Whether your speedwork is hill training, interval training, tempo running, or other variations on the speed theme, the advantage of training using an overload, or progressive, stage is that as you get tougher, you toughen the workouts. This approach provides a strong psychological "carrot" for the runner trying to peak for a specific race. After the long runs to develop endurance, after the fast runs to develop strength, you use a shot of speed training to fine-tune your speed.

HILL TRAINING

If you plan to run a hilly marathon, you need to do at least some of your training on hilly courses. Even if you live in the flattest of flat-lands, hills can be found if you search hard enough and are willing to climb into a car. The city of Chicago is flat, but several suburbs offer rolling hills. Runners in Jacksonville, Florida, preparing for the Gate River Run, a 15K, train over a 2-mile loop course that crosses two high bridges over the St. Johns River.

Increasing the angle of your treadmill to simulate uphill running is another option. Some high-tech treadmills can be adjusted to downhill. Downhill training is de rigueur if you are preparing for a marathon such as St. George (in Utah) or Boston. The St. George Marathon drops 2,600 feet, promising a fast toboggan ride—but not if you failed to train your quads to withstand the extra pounding they will absorb. Boston is hilly overall, but with more down than up: going from 490 feet above sea level in Hopkinton to 10 feet near the finish.

As part of my speed training, I often do hill repeats: starting with 3 × 400, adding one more repeat each week, and climaxing with 8 × 400. (The hill that ends near my driveway is about that long.) I run hard up, jog back down easy, then repeat.

Preparing for the Boston Marathon, I also run downhill repeats—typically, every second or third one. This is risky because the extra impact may cause an injury, but if you want to succeed at Boston, you need to prepare for the downs as well as the ups.

(continued)

Before Boston one year, Olympic marathoner Rod DeHaven prepared by placing a two-by-four under the rear of his treadmill. He
ran 2:12:41 at Boston.

   If you live in a hilly area and are training for a flat marathon such
as Chicago, the problem is the same, only in reverse. Find some
flat areas for your training.

NUMBERS

Blind application of any number-based training system can cause problems. One variable is weather. And *whether.* Whether it is cold or hot,
whether it is windy or rainy, can affect how fast or far you run during any
given workout. The number of miles you have run does not necessarily
reflect the quality of your training.

   Barry Brown, a top masters runner, commuted by air between offices
in Bolton Landing, New York, and Gainesville, Florida. Brown trained
with a heart monitor so he could measure the
relative intensity of his workouts, regardless

**The one factor
critical to your
taper is rest.**

of other variables. He once described to me
an interval workout featuring mile repetitions,
which he ran averaging 5:20 per mile in cool
weather in New York, then averaged 5:40 in hot
weather in Florida the following week. "The
intensity measured by my pulse rate was exactly the same," Barry told
me. "But if you just looked at the numbers in my diary, you would have
thought I was taking it easy in the second workout." Here is another example. A flight attendant with Delta Airlines lived in Boulder, Colorado;
was based in Atlanta, Georgia; and often flew to San Juan, Puerto Rico.
She worried about managing and measuring the intensity of her training schedule when shifting from altitude to sea level with accompanying

changes in temperature (and comfort), but sometimes you simply need to relax and not try to compare the numbers from one workout with those of the next or one week with the next. Those marvelous electronic devices we now use to measure our workouts can become traps if we fall slave to their numbers.

Fatigue, diet, and sleep can affect the intensity of your training. Monitoring intensity is probably the trickiest aspect of any training program, even for an experienced runner, and that is one reason a knowledgeable coach can help you shave minutes off your marathon time. Self-trained runners who are very motivated can get themselves in trouble too easily. If they train in a group, where group dynamics sometimes take precedence over good sense, they can encounter similar problems.

For these reasons, I do not recommend doing interval training—or any form of speedwork—year-round. Nevertheless, it is a type of training that lends itself well to progressing toward a specific goal.

TIME TO LOOK BACK

At various points during the premarathon buildup, I like to review what I am doing. Am I on schedule? Am I training too hard and do I need to back off? What level of fitness have I achieved, and how will that affect my pace in the marathon?

One year at the Chicago Marathon, a runner approached me and said that he would log on to the marathon training program on my website to see what he was supposed to run that day. After the workout, he would log back on to make sure he had done the workout correctly. You may be tempted to laugh, but what he achieved was positive reinforcement for his training. A lot of runners today who do not have easy access to good coaching use the Internet as their coach.

During any review, I decide only to decrease the level of my training; I never decide to increase it. If you think you are behind in your premarathon schedule, you need to either lower your performance expectations or choose another race later in the year.

One way to determine your fitness level is to enter a race over a well-established distance. It is easy enough to find a 5K or 10K to jump into, although the best test would be in a race closer in distance to the marathon. That is one reason I recommend running a half marathon midway through the training period. I do not like to race too often during my peak buildup for any major event, but particularly not before a marathon. To race properly, I find I need to rest several days before the race, and it takes me several days after it to recover. Before you know it, you have lost the equivalent of a week of productive training. For that reason, I try to limit any test races in the premarathon buildup to one a month.

Then there is what the group leaders who worked with me in the Chicago Marathon training class somewhat jokingly referred to as the triathlon problem. There was a late-summer triathlon in Chicago, and inevitably some individuals would want to enter both the tri and the marathon. "You can do both," we would usually tell them, "but it's difficult to do both well." We suggested they consider their priorities, establishing which race was more important and concentrating their main energy on that event. This might mean cutting back on the bike and swim training for the triathlon, then doing the tri as a hard workout rather than a race. Or do the marathon as an afterthought: 26 miles of low-pressure running without worrying about time.

Nevertheless, some racing is helpful. If you are a beginner, you will learn what it feels like to go to a starting line. Your time in test races can help you predict your marathon time and guide you in selecting a pace. But in making comparisons, beware of overconfidence. You may also need to make adjustments depending on conditions, including weather and the difficulty of the course.

ATOP THE MOUNTAIN

Eventually, if you have planned well, you will reach a peak in your training, the top of the mountain. Running becomes easier and less of a strain. You are able to finish your weekly long runs at the same pace you started, and you do not feel as tired or worn out the next day. If you are running speedwork on the track, your times are faster. You feel good. You look lean and mean. One of the best indicators of my fitness level was when my mother-in-law would look at me and say, "You're too skinny!" It was then that I knew I was in shape.

All of these signals offer positive feedback and will provide a psychological boost when you run your big race. If you know you're in shape, you are more likely to feel confident that you can achieve a peak performance. Mental strength may be as important as physical strength, but you achieve mental confidence by training yourself physically.

Most first-time marathoners train to reach a quick peak—that final 20-miler before the race. But if they are well coached, they will not try to achieve a peak performance in their first marathon; they will save that goal for future races.

Most experienced marathoners like to reach a peak, then hold that training level for 4 to 6 weeks. Once you get to the point at which you have the time and ability to run several 20-milers, you are more likely to achieve the peak performance you want. You will probably also chop minutes off the time you ran in your first marathon.

The final touch for any program designed to achieve peak performance is the taper, the gradual cutback of training immediately before the race. This is such an important subject that I have devoted an entire chapter to it. The one factor critical to your taper is rest, something many dedicated runners have trouble doing. You need to arrive at the starting line rested, refreshed, and ready to run, the three R's of peak performance. More on this to come.

HOW WELL DO MARATHONERS PREPARE?

How seriously do runners take their marathon preparation? More specific, once they decide to run a particular marathon, how many days and weeks do they devote to training? Judging from a quick survey I took of those following me on Twitter, runners do take their marathon training seriously. Three-quarters of those responding trained 18 weeks or more. (Eighteen weeks is the length of most of my marathon training programs.)

How long do runners train before a marathon?	
Less than 18 weeks	25%
18 weeks or more	36%
6 months or more	34%
A year or more	5%

Truth be told, these were runners who followed me on Twitter and thus already were predisposed to accept the numbers in my training programs. Also, a runner who maintains a high-mileage schedule so he or she can run three or four or more marathons a year certainly does not need to devote 18 weeks of specific training before each one. The take-home message from this survey is that, yes, we take our training seriously, and that includes the 5 percent who spend a year or more preparing for each of their marathon races.

16

Monitoring Your Heart Rate

Listen to the Beat

Among all of the world's workout areas, the trails of Indiana Dunes State Park remain my favorite. Often, I would train there several days a week, either solo or in company with longtime training partners from the Dunes Running Club. Typically, I would drive through the front entrance flashing my season pass, park, then head off quickly into the woods on Trail 2, mostly firm and flat, some of it boardwalk, a circular loop around a marsh near 3 miles long. For more miles, I would divert onto another loop, Trail 9, also near 3 miles, converting my circular loop into a figure-eight loop of a half-dozen miles with a few short hills to add variety to the workout. And for many workouts, I would choose a third loop, the so-called Ridge Trail that overlooks Lake Michigan, a roller-coaster ride that features a series of sharp ups and downs over soft sand and roots lurking like snakes to trip the unwary runner. What better way to raise a runner's heart rate?

And that was the purpose of a workout: to raise my heart rate to 90 percent of maximum, the lactate threshold zone where scientists tell us fine things happen to our bodies. But how do you measure such a workout? Distance is meaningless. Time is meaningless. One way to tell when you hit the 90 percent zone is by wearing a heart rate monitor.

Roy Benson, co-author with Declan Connolly of *Heart Rate Training*, offers a very simple explanation of why runners should consider adding a heart rate monitor to their collection of running gear: "It offers an objective measurement of how hard you're running."

Well said, Roy. Such monitors prove very useful if you plan to do speedwork. In Indiana Dunes State Park, where there are no mile markers, where the trees are so numerous and the leaves so thick during summer that GPS signals fail to penetrate the foliage, there is no way to tell how fast or far you are running. But with a heart rate monitor, you can rely on it to provide objective measurement on how hard you ran. You can even program it to beep when you

The faster we run, the faster beats our heart.

reach your 90 percent goal, and if your numbers decline during a slow-down (as in a fartlek workout), the watch will beep again to tell you once more to get going. You will have converted a traditional fartlek run into a *heartlek* run.

When I first used a heart rate to monitor my training, it meant wearing a belt around my chest with sensors capable of picking up the beat of my heart and giving me instant feedback. I could glance at my wrist and modify my pace based on the numbers I saw on my wristwatch. At the same time, this created a record. Back home after my run, I could see what my heart rate had been at 5-, 30-, and 60-second increments. Today's monitors, unsurprisingly, have more features, and the chest band no longer is a necessity. The sensors now have been miniaturized to measure heart rate from the wristwatch itself. Prices for devices (including heart rate monitors) that measure our workouts begin around $25 and peak somewhere around ten times that sum.

WHAT MONITORS MEASURE

The science behind heart rates is simple. When we are asleep, our heart beats slowly, just fast enough to match our slowed-down metabolism and keep us breathing. The minute we swing our feet out of bed, stand up, and start walking, the heart starts beating somewhat faster in order to send oxygen-rich blood to the now-demanding muscles. Eating breakfast causes another slight increase, because it takes energy to digest food. Sitting at a computer and typing, dealing with the stress of daily life, causes the heart to plateau at a level necessary to get us through the day.

But then, when we don running shoes and head out the door for our daily workout, we force the heart to beat faster. Our greedy muscles demand more and more oxygen. The faster we run, the faster beats our heart until it can no longer push more blood through the cardiovascular system. Our muscles scream "help," but no more help is coming. We have arrived at VO_2 max, the maximum volume of oxygen that the heart can offer our running muscles. We can hold at the 100 percent level only for a brief period of time: seconds, rather than minutes. Highly trained runners probably can continue running at max for somewhat longer than lesser-trained runners, but even they soon are forced to slow down. This causes the heart rate to drop, gradually at first until the muscles release their excessive demand for fuel, fuel, fuel; oxygen, oxygen, oxygen.

All this is easily measured on the wrist device that we purchased during our last visit to a specialty running store.

Roy Benson believes that the two most important uses of a heart rate monitor are to (1) keep you slow enough on the easy days, so that you can recover in time to run your best on the hard days, and (2) keep you from overtraining caused by pushing into what might be called the Dark Zone on those hard days.

Recently, I surveyed my online followers, asking: "Why use a heart monitor?" The results were interesting if not surprising. (Respondents were allowed to check more than one answer.)

It helps me analyze my training	32%
It teaches me to understand my body	15.3%
It helps me know my current fitness	15.3%
I use it to analyze race results	10.3%
It takes the guesswork out of training	7.7%
It helps me not to repeat mistakes	7.7%
It motivates me to train	6.4%
It allows me to plan my workouts	5.1%
It is fun to use	5.1%
It keeps me on pace during long runs	5.1%

I feel that all of the above are valid reasons. The one I like the most is the idea that heart monitors are "fun." While researching the first edition of this book, I used a monitor to learn how to do what coaches often recommend: "Listen to your body." I watched the numbers during workouts and analyzed my body's responses afterward.

Different runners value their heart rate monitors for different reasons. "The heart monitor is most useful to me during recovery runs and tempo workouts," says Jim Mulcahy from Glen Carbon, Illinois. "My heart rate floats a lot during easy runs: 148 one day; 160 the next, when I might be more tired. The numbers are the same during this training cycle versus last time, but I'm running 10 to 15 seconds a mile faster because I'm in better shape."

Martin Van Walsum from Carlisle, Massachusetts, believes his monitor helps him train more effectively: "Each run has a purpose. Knowing my heart rate is in the correct training zone helps keep me in the groove."

Benson and Connolly write: "The beauty of heart rate training is that it relies on a system (your cardiovascular system) that reflects your overall state of stress 24 hours a day, 365 days a year. It reflects when you're tired, overtrained, sick, cold, or hot and therefore can guide you in making changes to your plan. More important from an exercise point of view, it provides immediate and consistent feedback about your stress level."

"There are many reasons why an athlete's heart rate might vary from session to session," writes Pete Stock, a coach from Manchester, England. "They would include stress, lack of sleep, alcohol, caffeine, heat, hydration, and, of course, overtraining. As coaches, we can't instantly cure most of these for our athletes, but we can be aware of them and help the athlete understand their impact so they can deal with the consequences more effectively."

Let's consider how you might use a heart rate monitor to train. Benson and Connolly define the heart rate zones used in training as follows (the percentages quoted are the percentages of VO_2 max):

Heart Rate %	Effort Level	Pace	Goal
60%–75%	Easy	Slow	Endurance
75%–85%	Moderate	Moderate	Stamina
85%–95%	Difficult	Fast	Economy
95%–100%	Very hard	Sprint	Speed

Before you proceed to your running store to purchase your new gadget, a couple of caveats: First, the data you receive from any monitor is only as good as your ability to *interpret* that data. In using a heart monitor during marathons, I discovered that the numbers made sense only until I hit the wall. My heart was ticking along, but the rest of my body was not. As I slowed, my heart rate slowed to well below goal rate—except I was powerless to do anything about it. For me personally, checking heart rate was more useful during 5K and 10K races, where I could maintain a steady pace without crashing. But I have talked to many runners who have had success even at the longest distances. (The coach doesn't claim to know everything.)

Formulas do not work for everybody.

Second but equally important: the formulas that experts frequently offer for predicting maximum heart rate do not work for everybody. A common formula promoted by Dr. Kenneth H. Cooper is 200 minus half your age. I had a low pulse (30) and a low max (160), so the formulas never worked for me. At age 30, the formula said my max should have been 175. Not true. "It's okay to start with a formula," says Benson, "but common sense should immediately overrule numbers that cause you to run too slow or too fast, compared with effort level." A stress test under the supervision of a knowledgeable cardiologist or exercise scientist offers the best way to determine maximum heart rate so that you can use the percentages in the chart. Or, check your pulse rate at the end of a race at a relatively short distance, one in which you sprint for the finish line in the last 150 meters. If and when you hit VO_2 max, the numbers should plateau, meaning your heart is beating as hard as it can.

Frequently, I receive questions from runners puzzled by the results from their heart rate monitors. Typical would be, "My monitor tells me I'm running at 90 percent of max, but I'm moving at little more than a jog." Invariably, the reason is because the runner does not know his or her maximum heart rate. That included Megan Leahy, the former member of my cross-country team.

One day I took Megan to the high school track for a workout and asked her to wear my monitor while she did a series of interval quarters. Her heart rate spiked at 240! I was ready to dial 911, but it was an example of how varied healthy human beings can be when it comes to body functions.

To get an accurate idea of your VO_2 max, Roy Benson suggests the following eight-lap test you can do on a standard 400-meter track. Here is what to do each of the eight laps.

1. Walk at a normal pace.
2. Walk at a marching pace.
3. Jog at your slowest pace.
4. Run at an easy "conversational" pace.
5. Run hard enough so that talking becomes difficult.
6. Run hard enough so that talking is no longer possible.
7. Run faster and faster on the final 2 laps.
8. Break into an all-out sprint. Kick it home.

That's not easy to do. You almost need to be track trained, familiar with speedwork, to be able to sprint all-out in that final lap and push yourself to VO_2 max. To find out whether you succeeded in hitting VO_2 max, check your wristwatch afterward. During the final 60 to 90 seconds, your numbers should have plateaued. The heart can't pump blood to the muscles any faster. From that point forward, you can use that data to follow a training program based on heart rate.

As an example, here is my Advanced 1 marathon converted into an HR program using the percentages for Easy, Moderate, Difficult, and Very Hard. You can compare the numbers to the regular Advanced 1 program shown on page 328. I created this Heart Rate program more for fun than hoping some of you might precisely follow it. Thus rather than following the program precisely, use it as a guide in learning about your body, perhaps designing a program for yourself.

Marathon: Advanced 1 (Heart Rate)

Week	Mon	Tue	Wed	Thu	Fri	Sat	Sun
1	3-mile 60%	5-mile 75%	3-mile 65%	3 × hill 90%	Rest 0%	5-mile 80%	10-mile 65%
2	3-mile 60%	5-mile 75%	3-mile 65%	30 min. tempo 80%	Rest 0%	5-mile 70%	11-mile 65%
3	3-mile 60%	6-mile 75%	3-mile 65%	4 × 800 90%	Rest 0%	6-mile 80%	8-mile 65%
4	3-mile 60%	6-mile 75%	3-mile 65%	35 min. tempo 80%	Rest 0%	6-mile 80%	13-mile 65%
5	3-mile 60%	7-mile 75%	3-mile 65%	5 × 800 90%	Rest 0%	7-mile 70%	14-mile 65%
6	3-mile 60%	7-mile 75%	3-mile 65%	5 × 800 90%	Rest 0%	7-mile 80%	10-mile 65%
7	3-mile 60%	8-mile 75%	3-mile 65%	5 × hill 90%	Rest 0%	7-mile 80%	16-mile 65%
8	3-mile 60%	8-mile 75%	3-mile 65%	40 min. tempo 80%	Rest 0%	8-mile 70%	17-mile 65%
9	3-mile 60%	9-mile 75%	3-mile 65%	6 × 800 90%	Rest 0%	Rest 0%	Half 100%
10	3-mile 60%	9-mile 75%	3-mile 65%	6 × hill 90%	Rest 0%	9-mile 80%	19-mile 65%
11	4-mile 60%	10-mile 75%	4-mile 60%	45 min. tempo 80%	Rest 0%	10-mile 70%	20-mile 65%
12	4-mile 60%	6-mile 75%	4-mile 65%	7 × 800 90%	Rest 0%	6-mile 80%	12-mile 65%
13	4-mile 60%	10-mile 75%	4-mile 65%	7 × hill 90%	Rest 0%	10-mile pace	20-mile 65%
14	5-mile 60%	5-mile 75%	5-mile 65%	45 min. tempo 80%	Rest 0%	6-mile 70%	12-mile 65%
15	5-mile 60%	10-mile run	5-mile 65%	8 × 800 90%	Rest 0%	10-mile 80%	20-mile 65%
16	5-mile 60%	8-mile 75%	5-mile 65%	6 × hill 90%	Rest 0%	4-mile 80%	12-mile 65%
17	4-mile 60%	6-mile 75%	4-mile 65%	30 min. tempo 80%	Rest 0%	4-mile 70%	8-mile 65%
18	3-mile 50%	4 × 400 60%	2-mile 50%	Rest 0%	Rest 0%	2-mile 50%	Marathon 80%

17

The Magic Taper

For the Final 3 Weeks,
Do Next to Nothing

After months and months of training—after the steady buildup of weekly miles and strings of long runs on weekends—the big event is near. Many questions spring to mind: What do you do the last few weeks before the marathon? How do you prepare yourself physically and mentally? How much should you rest? How do you cut back on training? How long should you taper?

In the critical, final weeks just prior to the race, too many marathoners make a serious mistake. They fail to use one key ingredient in any training system, one that is mentioned many times in this book:

Rest!

David L. Costill, PhD, of the Human Performance Laboratory at Ball State University in Muncie, Indiana, believes that runners often train too hard in the weeks immediately preceding a marathon. "They feel they need one last butt-busting workout and end up tearing themselves down," he once told me.

That probably was truer two decades ago, before the first edition of this book and before coaches and runners finally figured out the secrets to success in this quirky sport of ours. In past years, many runners failed to taper much more than a week, even for major marathons. But by the 1990s and leading into the new millennium, more and more marathons provided training classes for the convenience of their runners. Increasing numbers of coaches began to serve the large pool of new runners. And with the explosion of training advice on the Internet, especially for beginning runners, the word has gotten out: You do need to cut back on your training for several weeks to obtain a peak performance. In his research with swimmers, Dr. Costill noticed that they often set PRs when they tapered as much as 3 to 6 weeks before an event.

Swimmers, he felt, performed better when undertrained. In one study, Dr. Costill tapered a group of track athletes 3 weeks before a race. During this test period, they ran only 2 easy miles daily. Two problems developed. First, psychological tests showed that the runners worried about losing conditioning and became anxious. This is common; I see it all the time among participants in my online boards. Second, in a preliminary 5000-meter (5K) trial, the runners—apparently so well rested that they misjudged their abilities—started off too fast and faded at the end. But in a subsequent trial, the runners did pace themselves better and ran their best times.

> **You do need to cut back on your training for several weeks.**

Dr. Costill eventually concluded that runners could best achieve success in long-distance running by preparing far in advance: "Base is important. Runners need to start their marathon training early enough so that they can afford to taper 2 or 3 weeks before the event. You need to realize that it is the training you do months before—rather than weeks before—that spells success."

That is a message we all should heed, but the drive that pushes us to success often pushes us to train too hard at the end. This is particularly true of seasoned marathoners. They become comfortable with their regular training routines—whether it is 40, 50, 60, or more weekly miles—and do not want to cut back.

You may not know what to do with the extra time. And you do not want to give up your long Sunday run with friends, even the last weekend before the marathon. Then there is the problem of diet. If you cut down on the number of miles you run, you may also need to cut the number of calories you eat if you do not want to gain weight. And although many marathoners may believe that rest could benefit their performance in a particular marathon, they are afraid of the effect of 2 or 3 weeks' rest on their overall conditioning.

CHANGING HABITS

Nevertheless, if you want to run well in the marathon, you must change your habits in five areas in those final weeks leading up to the race.

1. LOWER TOTAL MILEAGE

Many of us are slaves to our training logs. We find security in the consistency with which we run week after week, month after month, recording a steady succession of miles covered. That's fine, since consistent training brings results, but for the last 2 to 3 weeks before the marathon, mileage does not count. In fact, high mileage may hinder your performance.

Scientific research shows that cutting back on training boosts leg muscle power and reduces lactic acid production. Hard workouts, however, can produce nagging injuries and deplete leg muscles of their key fuel for running—glycogen.

How much should you cut mileage? That is a tough question because all of us are different, and our goals differ. As a general rule, I recommend cutting total mileage during the last 3 weeks by at least 50 percent. (Later in this chapter, I present specific directions for how to do this.)

2. MODIFY THE FREQUENCY OF YOUR RUNS

The simplest way to cut total mileage is to reduce the number of times you train. When I was training at the elite level and running twice a day, I cut my mileage by eliminating one of those daily workouts the last 10 days before a race.

You may not train twice daily, but if you follow a hard/easy pattern in your training, you have a similar option. Just eliminate the easy days. Instead of running an easy 3-miler on your in-between days, do not run at all. Take a day off. Your body will be able to recover more fully from the hard workouts, and you will not lose any conditioning.

3. CUT DISTANCE, THOUGH NOT INTENSITY

Research also suggests that you need to continue to train at or near race pace on the hard days. At McMaster University in Hamilton, Ontario, a group led by Duncan MacDougall, PhD, compared different ways of tapering for well-trained runners who averaged 45 to 50 miles a week. For the taper week, some athletes did not run, others ran 18 to 19 miles at an easy pace, and another group cut their mileage but continued running fast. The researchers decided a taper that includes small amounts of fast running is superior to slow, easy miles.

The McMaster group also worked with runners training for a 10K race who started their tapers with 5 × 500 meters at race pace, then progressively eliminated one 500 for each of the next 5 days, ending with a rest day. (In other words: 5 × 500, 4 × 500, 3 × 500, 2 × 500, 1 × 500, rest.)

Dr. MacDougall comments: "We still don't know what the optimal tapering plan actually is, but we do know that if you're going to be tapering for a week or so, it's important to keep the intensity of your workouts fairly high as you cut back drastically on your mileage."

Translated to the marathon, this would mean maintaining the pace of your runs but cutting their distance. A hard 8-mile run would become a 6-mile run at the beginning of the taper, then later get cut to 4 or 2. But you should keep the pace near the comfortable one you've used for most of your training. In speed workouts, cut the number of repetitions, similar to the McMaster taper.

4. STOP LIFTING

If you are a frequent visitor to the weight room and lift weights two or three times a week or more, that is good for your physical fitness and overall health, but you need to cut back on this discipline, too, as marathon day nears.

Certainly during the last 3 weeks before the marathon, you need to match what you do on the roads with what you do in the gym. No heavy lifting. Fewer repetitions. Grab your towel and head to the shower feeling exhilarated, not exhausted.

In fact, a 3-week taper for lifters may not be enough, particularly for those who did not spend a lot of time in the gym before becoming runners. Taper your lifting 6 weeks out, at the time you hit peak running mileage. That will decrease the chance of injury either running or lifting.

Eliminate junk food from your diet during taper week.

5. LOWER THAT CALORIE LEVEL

Finally, watch what you eat. If you are running less, you are also burning fewer calories. This could mean you gain a pound or so—no big deal, unless you also fill in your spare time by making extra trips to the fridge.

Watch your intake for the first 3 days of the marathon week to avoid weight gain, then the next 3 days eat more than your normal intake, with the emphasis on carbohydrates.

To keep from piling on extra pounds, eliminate junk food from your diet during taper week. Get rid of the soft drinks and sweets that you may have used to boost calorie intake during regular training. Rely on complex carbohydrates instead—potatoes, apples, pasta, bread, and so on.

EXPERIENCE COUNTS

Knowing precisely how to modify your training before a marathon takes experience. Even for seasoned marathoners, it may take a few bad starts before finding a specific routine that works. There are too many variables in the equation: how long you might have prepared for a particular long race, how effective your training has been, whether you enter the closing stages undertrained or overtrained, and how confident you are.

TAPERING TIME

Before a marathon, how much should you taper? For some low-key races, I might run right up to the point where disaster lurks around the corner, tapering only the last 3 days. There also was a period during the popularity of so-called carbo-loading, when I would do my final 20-miler 1 week out, then after a 3-day depletion phase (low carb) do a loading phase for 3 days (high carb) leading to the marathon. Eventually (listening to the scientists), I decided that did not work and settled on 10 days as perfect for me.

Notice I said "for me." I was a high-mileage runner (100 miles weekly), and I now suggest 3 weeks for those following my training programs, again listening to the scientists. This survey suggests that not everybody who follows me on Twitter accepts my advice. But I am the first to admit that we are all different, as suggested by the survey results.

Tapering Before Marathon	Percentages
3 days before marathon	3%
1 week before marathon	32%
10 days before marathon	33%
3 weeks before marathon	28%

A good coach who is familiar with your abilities and training patterns can tell you how to taper. A coach who has worked with you on a daily basis can tell you precisely how to modify your training for the final countdown. Although I frequently get involved in writing training schedules to be offered online and in books, one single program cannot be expected to fit all runners. Nevertheless, here's my spin on the last 3 weeks before the big race.

THREE FOR THE MONEY

Three weeks (21 days) before the race and after your final 20-miler, start to cut back. You know what to do; do it! For all practical purposes, your marathon training is over. Avoid the trap of thinking that 1 additional week of training just might get you in really good shape. It is more likely to injure you or lower your resistance so you are at risk of catching a cold or the flu—a big liability when you have a race to run.

This is particularly important if illness or injury forced you to miss a week or two of training during your ramp-up to the marathon. You do not—repeat, do not—want to make up that lost mileage now.

In almost all my marathon training programs, I prescribe the final 20-miler on the Saturday or Sunday before the 3-week taper begins. On successive weekends, the long run drops from 20 to 12 to 8 miles, with the marathon falling on the fourth weekend. The more I work with both beginning and even experienced runners, the more comfortable I become with this pattern. Most runners, at any level, will benefit from a slight decrease in their weekly mileage, to about 75 percent the first tapering week. The runner who ran 40 miles last week should cut back to about 30 miles. An easy way to cut total mileage is to convert 1 or 2 of your easy days into rest days. Change one or two others into half workouts, decreasing your distance. But do not cut intensity or pace yet. You

You know what to do; do it!

can cut the number of repeats during speed workouts, for example, but do not necessarily run them slower.

TWO FOR THE SHOW

Two weeks (14 days) out: If you did not significantly cut mileage last week, do so now. You need at least this much time to taper. In my peak years, I tapered exactly 10 days before marathons. Now that I am older and wiser, I take more time. If you feel you must run a 20-miler 2 weeks before the race, it should be your final workout at this distance. In my 12-week Boston Bound program for runners qualified for and running the Boston Marathon, the final 20-miler is 2 weeks and 1 day out (Boston being on a Monday). But runners with a BQ can handle that short a taper.

With several thousand people around you on race day, you are not going to get lost.

If you did cut your mileage to 75 percent the week before, now you should cut it to nearly 50 percent of your normal mileage. The marathoner who normally runs 40 miles a week should run maybe 20 miles this week.

But do not reduce your pace yet. You do not want to forget too soon what it feels like to train at near-marathon pace.

Remember that along with the decreased mileage, you will be burning fewer calories. So if you are worried about gaining a pound or two, cut back on your intake of "empty" calories.

ONE TO GET READY

One week (7 days) before your big race, if you have resisted the idea of cutting your mileage before, you definitely need a reality check. Cut it out—now! Even another-lap-around-the-park zealots will concede that maybe a little rest is helpful at this point. Do you really believe running 20 miles the final Sunday before your race is going to help you? Were you born in Kenya? And I'm not sure even the Kenyans are out banging the roads that much the weekend before. At one point in my running career, I felt comfortable floating through a final 20, but I'm older and wiser now.

Begin carbo-loading 7 days in advance. Stick with a high-carbohydrate diet throughout the week. You do not need to eat spaghetti all 7 days; focusing on fruits, vegetables, and grains will keep you near 60 percent carbs even if you have lean meat as a main course. The secret meal of the Kenyans is ugali, what the Italians call polenta, a cornmeal porridge. It allows them to push their regular diets to near 70 percent carbohydrates.

If you have not eliminated between-meal junk snacks, what is the matter with you? Have you not been paying attention? Do it now! This is also the week to eliminate not merely hard training but any sort of training. There is no room in your training plan for hard, fast, or long runs. Forget them. If you run anything at or near race pace, do not run far.

Now is also not—repeat, *not*—the time to cross-train. One problem is that people sometimes use these lower-mileage weeks to do something else equally stressful. Do not hang out in the gym. Do not go for a bike ride. Do not swim. Do not hike in the mountains. Do not pass Go. You will not be handed $200, or an equivalent fast time. Use the extra time to catch up on family and work responsibilities.

TIME TO GO

Three days remain. For the final 3 days of the countdown, I shift to almost total rest. Notice I said "almost." During the final 3 days, I rest 2, run 1. This is my usual premarathon pattern:

Three days before is a day off.
Two days before is a day off.

One day before, I may do some light jogging and perhaps a few
   strides, particularly if I have traveled a long distance to the race.

Strides are controlled sprints at race pace. I do a couple of miles of easy
running to loosen up, particularly if I traveled to the race by car or plane.
Strides are short: 150 meters at the most. Soft surfaces are best. Instead of
jogging between strides, I'll walk. Before Boston, staying in a hotel near
the finish line on Boylston Street, I run a couple of blocks to the Charles
River and do my strides on the grass beside the bike path. In Chicago,
there's plenty of grass in Grant Park near the start of the race. In midtown
New York, head to Central Park. Most runners find prerace training areas
without much prodding.

If possible, travel at least 2 days before the race, not the day before,
especially if travel fatigues you. One rule of thumb is to arrive 1 day early
for every time zone crossed, but that is not easy to do if your destination
race is in Australia or South Africa or Argentina.

THE FINAL 24 HOURS

The important point to remember about the last 24 hours is that if you
have prepared properly, nothing much you do on this day—except what
you eat and drink—will have much effect on your race. Mental preparation is probably more important than physical preparation at this point.

One way to pass time the day before the race is to hang out at the expo,
an important part of the marathon experience. But do not spend all day
on your feet, particularly given the hard concrete in most expo halls. If
you want to chat with your friends, do it in your room or sitting in soft
chairs in the hotel lobby.

Another option is touring the course. Some runners feel it is important
to see the course in advance so they know what to expect. But having
been in the running business this long as both participant and reporter, I
have either run most of the major courses or ridden them in press trucks.

I do not need to see them one more time, particularly if it means committing myself to sitting for several hours on a bus. Touring race courses was more important to me when I was younger and anticipating running in the lead, but with several thousand people around you on race day, you are not going to get lost.

To me, the hills always seem steeper and the miles longer when you are riding over them rather than running them. If there are key points of a course I feel I need to check out—such as a series of hills—I might make an effort to see them, but usually I am content to wait until race day.

Wherever or whatever you eat, your last meal needs to be high in carbohydrates. But do not overeat, thinking more is better. Even though the second and third helpings are free, do not necessarily avail yourself of them. Eat a normal-size meal and drink what you usually drink. In the past, I noticed a lot of runners walking around expos with water bottles in their hands. I see that less often now, so I suspect that the drink-until-you-drown approach to hydration is past its time. Most experts advise against beer because it is a diuretic, but if you are used to having an occasional beer or glass of wine with your meal and you think it will relax you, it probably will.

More important than the night before the race is the night before the night before.

Research at Ball State University suggests that eating two small meals 4 hours apart the night before the race may be better than eating one larger meal. Logistically, that used to be difficult to do, but with so many energy drinks and bars on the market, carbo-loading has become easier. Dr. Costill suggests that having a high-carbohydrate snack just before going to bed may help ensure a full supply of glycogen in your muscles. Avoid soft drinks with caffeine, which may keep you awake. My caffeine limit is normally one cup of coffee or one soft drink, but I will not have even that the night before a marathon.

With or without caffeine in my system, I may sleep fitfully or awaken in the middle of the night. This used to worry me; it no longer does. I thought I was losing energy by lying awake in bed, but as long as you're horizontal, you are still getting rest. More important than the night before the race is two nights before the race. For a Sunday race, make certain you sleep well on Friday, and do not worry about Saturday.

One final item in my premarathon countdown: I know this sounds obsessive, but I always pin my number on my singlet before I go to bed. I also bring extra safety pins in case there are not enough in the race packet. With my singlet so pinned—and I will try it on to make certain I have not pinned the front to the back—I position it on a chair, along with my shorts, warmup clothes, and any other gear, with my shoes (socks inside) under the chair and pointing in the right direction, as though I were seated there sort of like a fireman having his boots ready before sliding down the pole. I once felt somewhat foolish doing this, but I have talked to enough runners to realize that I am not alone in this practice. Or maybe most have read a previous edition of this book and picked up my eccentric habits.

Be sure to check to make sure you have all of the necessary gear before you leave home. A friend of mine once confessed to putting on what he thought were his shoes the morning of the Boston Marathon only to discover he had packed his wife's running shoes. Same model; not the same size. Savvy marathoners also carry their shoes on the plane just in case the airline loses their bags.

When it comes to the marathon, you do not want to leave anything to chance.

TAPERING FOR THE HALF

Although I suggest a 3-week taper for the marathon, tapering that much for a half marathon or other less-than-26 race would be overkill. My half marathon training programs last 12 weeks, compared with 18 for the marathon. Training programs for 5K and 10K races are 8 weeks long. At the risk of stating the obvious, you can train adequately for shorter races in less time, and you also need less tapering time.

A week's taper should be adequate for a half marathon, even for beginning runners running their first race at any distance. Two or 3 days' taper would be sufficient rest for races shorter than that.

How long you taper depends partially on your previous racing experience and fitness level. If you are running a 10K or half as an afterthought en route to a marathon, you may not even want to taper. Treat the race as a training run: a day or two off before, a day or two off after.

Here is the final-week taper for my Novice 1 half-marathon program.

Week	Mon	Tue	Wed	Thur	Fri	Sat	Sun
12	Rest	3-mile run	2-mile pace	2-mile run	Rest	Rest	Half mara-thon

18

The Distance Runner's Diet

Fuel Your Body with the
Proper Foods

Can better nutrition create better athletes? When I asked that question some years ago of Ann C. Grandjean, EdD, director of the International Center for Sports Nutrition in Omaha, Nebraska, she offered a one-word answer: "Genetics!" What Dr. Grandjean meant was that great athletes are born with the ability to succeed, a gift of good genes that allows them—when properly trained and fed—to run and jump and throw faster and higher and farther than their less genetically gifted opponents. In suggesting better nutrition for long-distance runners, she knew that sports nutritionists cannot promise you success—but at least you will not fail because of poor nutrition and not be left wondering how much better you could be.

How important is good nutrition? Frederick C. Hagerman, PhD, of Ohio University in Athens, led off a conference in Columbus, Ohio, on nutrition for the marathon and other endurance sports prior to the men's Olympic marathon trials by saying that the second most important question asked by athletes is "What should I eat to make me stronger, better, and faster for my sport?" (The most important question, he said, is "How do I train?") Dr. Hagerman claimed that too many athletes had no idea how to eat properly to maximize their performance. These athletes also failed to realize that performance actually starts with the stomach, not with training.

There are three important areas of the distance runner's diet. One is overall nutrition, the ability to maintain high energy levels during training. The second is prerace nutrition, what you eat in the last few days before running to ensure a good performance. Third is what you consume before and during the race itself to make sure that you maximize performance—and get to the finish line on your own two feet. This chapter covers the first two, training nutrition and prerace nutrition. Your body's needs during the race are covered in Chapter 21, "Drinking on the Run."

THE RIGHT FUEL

Let's talk about why diet (i.e., finding the right fuel) is so important to your performance, not to mention your health. When you run long distances, your energy requirements increase. In an article on endurance exercise in the journal *The Physician and Sportsmedicine*, authors Walter R. Frontera, MD, and Richard P. Adams, PhD, said, "During sustained exercise such as marathon running, total body energy requirements increase 10 to 20 times above resting values." Runners need to eat more of the proper foods to fuel their muscles. They also need to drink more, particularly in warm weather.

At a sports nutrition conference in Columbus, Linda Houtkooper, PhD, a registered dietitian at the University of Arizona at Tucson, made it clear that endurance athletes in particular should get most of their calories from carbohydrates, preferably wholesome fruits, vegetables, and whole grains.

Carbs have been recognized as the preferred fuel for the endurance athlete because they are easy to digest and easy to convert into energy. Carbohydrates convert quickly into glucose (a form of sugar that circulates in the blood) and glycogen (the form of glucose stored in muscle tissue and the liver). Proteins can convert into glucose/glycogen, but at a greater energy cost. Fats can get easily stored as body fat. The body can normally store about 2,000 calories' worth of carbohydrate (glycogen) in the muscle, enough for maybe 20 miles of running.

No argument there. The only problem is that with 35,000 items in the supermarket, marathon runners sometimes need help determining which foods are highest in quality carbohydrates (as opposed to refined sugar).

Endurance athletes in particular should get most of their calories from carbohydrates.

Unless you plan to eat spaghetti three meals a day (and even pasta contains 13 percent protein and 4 percent fat), you may need to start reading labels.

Dr. Houtkooper explained that the body requires at least forty nutrients that are classified into six nutritional components: proteins, carbohydrates, fats, vitamins, minerals, and water. "These nutrients cannot be made in the body and so must be supplied from solid or liquid foods," she says. Plus, food contains a myriad of phytochemicals and other bioactive compounds that promote good health. She listed six categories that form the fundamentals of a nutritionally adequate food selection plan (in descending order of importance): fruits, vegetables, grains, lean meats/legumes/nuts, low-fat milk products, and fats/sweets.

The recommendations for a healthy diet suggest that carbohydrates (55 percent) should be the foundation of each meal, with some protein (15 percent) as the accompaniment and a little bit of healthy fat (30 percent) to add flavor and satiety. That is the gold standard and one that I offer to runners asking me questions online about nutrition. But all carbohydrates are not created alike. There are simple and complex carbs, sugars, and starches; refined and unprocessed carbs; "good carbs" and "bad carbs." The topic is very complex.

Refined carbs include sugar, honey, jam, sweets, and soft drinks. Nutritionists recommend that refined, simple sugars make up only 10 percent of your diet because they are nutrient poor, offering minimal vitamins and minerals. You want to concentrate your diet on wholesome "quality carbohydrates" from fruits, vegetables, whole-grain bread and pasta, and beans/legumes.

Endurance athletes in particular benefit from a carbohydrate-rich plant-based diet because of the muscle glycogen they burn each day that needs to be replenished. You need to aim for more total carbohydrates than people who fail to exercise. You can eat (in fact, may need to eat) more total calories without experiencing weight gain. The average male runner training for a marathon and running 25 to 30 miles a week probably needs a daily caloric intake near 3,000 to maintain muscle glycogen stores. As your mileage climbs beyond that, you need to eat more and more food, not less. In all honesty, this is why a lot of runners run and why they train for marathons. Their common motto is "I love to eat." But a word of caution: Some runners are "sedentary athletes." They may run hard for an hour, then sit the rest of the day. They may fail to burn as many calories as they think they do; then they overeat and end up gaining weight.

CARBOHYDRATES FOR PERFORMANCE

"Athletes who restrict carbs pay the price: 'dead legs' and an inability to exercise at their best," says sports nutritionist Nancy Clark. If you routinely train hard 4 to 6 days a week, carbs should be the foundation of each meal. Here are the International Olympic Committee's research-based carb recommendations for an optimal sports diet:

(continued)

Amount of exercise daily	Grams of carbs per pound of body weight	Grams of carbs per kilogram of body weight
1 hour moderate exercise	2.5 to 3 g	5 to 7 g
1 to 3 hours endurance exercise	2.5 to 4.5 g	6 to 10 g
4 to 5 hours extreme exercise	3.5 to 5.5 g	8 to 12 g

For a 150-pound runner who trains hard 1 hour a day and remains somewhat active the rest of the day, the target intake should be 375 to 450 grams of carbohydrate per day. That's at least 90 grams (360 calories) of carbohydrates per meal and 50 grams (200 calories) of carbs at each of two snacks. This is more carbs than in the ever-popular (low-carb) breakfast protein shake blended with a few berries, a lunchtime spinach salad, and a dinner with a pile of broccoli and chicken but no rice. Here's what 375 grams of carbohydrate looks like (without the protein and fat that balances the diet):

Breakfast: 1 cup dry oats (50 g) + 1 banana (25 g) + 1 Tbsp honey (15 g)

Lunch: 2 slices whole-wheat bread (46 g) + 1 can lentil soup (60 g)

Snack: ⅓ cup raisins (40 g) + 1 Tbsp dark chocolate chips (10 g)

Dinner: 1.5 cups cooked brown rice (65 g) + 14-ounce bag frozen broccoli (20 g)

Snack: 8 ounces vanilla Greek yogurt (20 g) + 1 granola bar (30 g)

Although I am sure many of you are rolling your eyes right now and thinking, "I could never eat that many carbs without getting fat," this is an appropriate carb intake, believe it or not, and these 1,500 carb-calories can fit into your day's 2,500+ calorie budget. I invite you to be curious and experiment. How much better can you train with an appropriate carb intake? Let's find out.

THE DISASTER DIET

The ageless Atkins diet and various other low-carb fad diets (like paleo or ketogenic) offer little more than a trap for distance runners. This is true of almost any weight-loss diet that limits carbohydrate intake. Go on one of these fad diets and you may experience a sudden reduction in weight, as measured by your bathroom scale. This weight loss, often dramatic, provides an instant boost to the dieter's ego and may cause the individual to stay on the diet and continue to lose weight. That is good. But the instant loss is artificial, since the shift in the protein/carbohydrate ratio causes the body to lose fluids.

There are no magic diets when it comes to weight loss.

For each 1 ounce of carbs the body stores as glycogen, the body also stores about 3 ounces of water. When you deplete those carbs, you lose water weight. That is not the greatest prerace strategy, since dehydration can be a danger for those training for a marathon, and particularly during the marathon itself. Add to that the discomfort caused by constipation, a side effect of a low-carb diet, which typically contains an inadequate supply of fiber-rich fruits, veggies, and whole grains.

Someone who is clinically obese can easily lose 5 to 10 pounds within a few weeks simply through this process of dehydration. But that person will continue to lose weight and maintain that weight loss only if he or she restricts calorie intake. There are no magic diets when it comes to weight loss. It is calories in versus calories burned, and the weight-loss regimens that work best are those that create a small but sustainable calorie deficit. For example, one runner eliminated two cans of cola a day (300 calories) and lost 30 pounds in a year because of that simple, sustainable dietary change. Just cutting 100 calories a day theoretically leads to 10 pounds of fat loss a year in a runner who has excess fat to lose.

Some high-mileage athletes actually may need to supplement their diets with high-carbohydrate 100 percent fruit juices to ensure sufficient energy for their daily runs. But you also need more protein, says Liz Applegate, PhD, a professor at the University of California at Davis, and the author of *Eat Smart, Play Hard*. Dr. Applegate suggests that runners training for a marathon need a minimum of 70 grams of protein a day—more if you're a high-mileage trainer. Most important, she advises, you need that protein distributed evenly throughout the day, including soon after you exercise, particularly after workouts longer than 10 miles.

"Eating a bagel or candy bar to quickly restore the calories you burned is not enough," argues Dr. Applegate. "Better would be a chug of chocolate milk or a tuna sandwich and piece of fruit. For the recovery meal, you need to eat three to four times more calories of carbohydrates than of protein (a ratio of about 3 or 4 grams carbohydrate to 1 gram protein). The longer the run, and the sooner you plan to train again, the more important this becomes." Following the 4-to-1 rule is particularly important after long runs. If you plan to use an energy bar before or after a long run, you need to read the label, says Dr. Applegate, since some bars contain mostly carbohydrates, while others may include large amounts of protein. You want a bar that offers both carbs and protein. The same goes for protein shakes. You want a fruit smoothie with some added protein; not just a low-carb, high-protein shake, Also note that recovery can start with your prerun meal. Hence, you want to eat carbs and protein both before and after you exercise.

CARBS RULE

Nevertheless, carbohydrates still rule. Serious runners may need about 3 to 4 grams of carbs per pound of ideal body weight. If you are a lean, mean 150 pounds, this comes to about 450 to 600 grams per day. Eating such a high-carbohydrate diet allows you to continuously restock your muscles with glycogen, the fuel that is as important in training as it is in racing. Because of the number of miles you run, you can also afford a somewhat higher ratio of simple versus complex carbohydrates in your diet—preferably in the form of 100 percent fruit juice and fresh fruit, though gummy bears and marshmallows will also fuel your muscles (minus the investment in good health).

Here is where I part company with the popular low-carb diets (Atkins, South Beach, the Zone, and so forth) that suggest food ratios near 40 percent carbohydrates, 30 percent protein, and 30 percent fat. Or the high-fat keto diet with less than 50 grams (200 calories) of carbs a day. People do lose weight following low-carb diets, although researchers suggest it is mainly because in following this regimen, they also cut calorie intake. On the other hand, plant-based diets, according to the Academy of Nutrition and Dietetics, are a healthy option for athletes interested in eliminating meat from their daily meals. When it comes to losing weight, all nutritionists agree that the best approach is to combine diet and exercise, and eat just a little less to create a small but effective and sustainable calorie deficit. And even this may not be enough if dieting causes a metabolism slowdown.

FOODS RICH IN CARBOHYDRATES

The traditional prerace meal for marathoners is pasta. With a wife of Italian American origin, I reap the culinary benefits of a tradition

(continued)

that literally demands frequent doses of pasta. But spaghetti (or macaroni or other forms of pasta) every day can become boring, particularly when you're trying to eat a carbohydrate-based diet every day to support your hard training. Fortunately, there are many foods you can eat to guarantee that your diet is high in carbohydrates, both during training and before races.

Nancy Clark's Sports Nutrition Guidebook lists the following carbohydrate-rich foods.

FRUITS
Apples
Bananas
Dates
Dried apricots
Oranges
Raisins

VEGETABLES
Broccoli
Carrots
Green beans
Peas
Tomato sauce
Winter squash

GRAINS, LEGUMES, AND POTATOES
Baked (sweet) potato
Beans (pinto, kidney, garbanzo, etc.)
Corn
Hummus
Lentils
Pasta, all shapes
Quinoa
Rice

BREADS, ROLLS, AND CRACKERS

Bagels
Bran and corn muffins
English muffins
Graham crackers
Matzo
Pancakes
Pita, wraps
Pretzels
Waffles
Whole-grain breads and rolls
Popcorn

BREAKFAST CEREALS

Cream of wheat
Granola
Grape-Nuts
Muesli
Oatmeal
Raisin bran

BEVERAGES

Apple cider
Cran-raspberry juice
Flavored milk
Fruit smoothie
Orange juice

SWEETS, SNACKS, AND DESSERTS

Cranberry sauce
Fig bars
Fruit yogurt
Honey

(continued)

> Maple syrup
> Strawberry jam
>
> Clark warns that some foods that runners assume are high in carbohydrates may have a high percentage of calories hidden in fat. These foods include croissants, Ritz crackers, thin-crust pizza, and granola. When in doubt, Clark advises, read the labels.

Running can be an effective fat-burning exercise (though burning fat differs from losing body fat, which requires a calorie deficit). You will burn approximately 100 calories a mile if you weigh around 150 pounds. If you weigh more, you burn more, which I suppose may be one of the few benefits of carrying a few extra pounds when you run. Nevertheless, run 36 miles (3,600 calories burned) and you can theoretically lose a pound of fat—assuming you do not replace those calories with hefty postrun meals. Follow my marathon training program and you will run approximately 500 miles over a period of 18 weeks. Theoretically, at least, you can lose 15 pounds by training for a marathon. This assumes that you do not increase your calorie consumption to meet your body's increased energy needs.

As your mileage climbs, you need to eat more and more food.

Some people seeking to finish their first marathon, however, are more than 15 pounds overweight—or they think they are—so they attempt to drop some additional pounds by dieting. To a certain extent, this is not a bad idea, assuming you choose your eating plan prudently. Those who follow a fad diet that lowers carbohydrate intake make a major mistake, because most of those programs fail to provide enough energy for endurance activities. Follow a low-carb diet, for example, and if you're eating 3,000 calories a day, you'll ingest much less than the 400 grams of carbohydrate recommended according to Dr. Applegate. "One problem," she says, "is that individuals following a low-carb diet Monday to Thursday start running out of energy by the weekend, when they're about to do their long run. They need to take a day off on Friday, not to rest from their running, but to rest from their diet. These low-carb runners either crash during the workout or binge on carbs to survive, which makes them feel guilty."

The aspects of most low-carb diets that Dr. Applegate likes is their emphasis on low-carb fruits and veggies, such as berries and leafy green vegetables, and protein. She feels that runners who graze on too many refined carbs (pretzels, bagels, jelly beans) and entirely avoid meats and other protein sources are not doing themselves any favors.

You do not need to patronize Italian restaurants to ensure an adequate supply of complex carbohydrates. I sometimes choose a Chinese restaurant because rice is also high in carbs. And Nancy Clark points out that you can get plenty of carbs in most American restaurants. If you eat soup (such as minestrone, bean, rice, or noodle), potatoes, breads, and vegetables along with your main dish and maybe enjoy a piece of apple cobbler off the dessert tray, you can end up eating more carbohydrates than fats or protein.

Or take your cue from the Kenyans, whose typical diet is ugali, a type of cornmeal porridge, also known as obusuma, nshima, mielepap, phutu, or sadza depending on where you land on the African continent. My Italian relatives call the meal polenta, but regardless of regional name, ugali is very high in carbohydrates, which allows Kenyan runners to maintain a 70 percent high-carb diet, a number that most Westerners would find difficult to match.

PREMARATHON NUTRITION

Pasta has become the ritual prerace feast for marathoners. No major marathon is without its night-before spaghetti dinner, which has assumed almost ceremonial aspects.

(continued)

The spaghetti dinner, of course, has more than a ceremonial purpose. We eat high-carbohydrate pasta to make sure our bodies have adequate glycogen, the fuel supply stored in the muscles that allows the most efficient form of energy metabolism. Although you could adapt to burning fat, fat metabolism requires more oxygen, and that limits performance when you are trying to surge up a hill or sprint to the finish line. The more glycogen you can store, the faster you can run for longer periods of time, because when muscle glycogen is depleted, muscles contract poorly. But a well-fueled athlete also needs a full supply of glycogen for the liver, a "processing station" that sends fuel through the bloodstream to the muscles and brain. So in addition to having your fuel tank to your hybrid car full, you need a fully charged battery. If you experience low blood sugar, your brain will lack fuel. You'll have trouble concentrating and focusing on the task at hand and instead wish you had never started this adventure. Bad mood, bad performance.

Various diets have been devised in an attempt to ensure maximum glycogen storage. Entire books have been written on the subject of sports nutrition, but premarathon eating is not that difficult. Simply concentrate on eating your standard carb-based training diet, and taper your training the final days before the marathon. For most endurance athletes who do follow a plant-based diet rich in grains, fruits, and vegetables, carbo-loading requires minimal changes to your regular daily eating routine; the bigger changes are in your training routine. This is good because you do not want to subject your system to any radical shifts just when you are about to run 26 miles. By running less, you allow your muscles the time they need to replenish depleted glycogen stores.

If you are racing out of town, you may want to take along some snacks to eat between the pasta dinner and the race the next morning. Graham crackers, energy bars, and vanilla wafers can be particularly useful, especially if you are competing in a foreign country where you're not accustomed to the food.

MEASURE YOUR FOODS

I do not spend a lot of time agonizing over what I eat, but on one occasion when a dietitian evaluated my diet, I averaged 12 percent protein, 19 percent fat, and 68 percent carbohydrates over a typical 3-day period. Fifty-two percent of my total calories came from complex carbohydrates, and 16 percent were from simple carbohydrates. (Dr. Applegate might argue that I was somewhat deficient in protein and a bit high on sweets, but I later corrected that in my diet.) A good target for most runners is about 55 percent to 65 percent carbs, 10 percent to 15 percent protein, and 20 percent to 30 percent fat. If you want to analyze your diet, use apps such as MyFitnessPal, LoseIt! or SparkPeople.com. When evaluating your daily food intake, be sure to serve yourself your normal portion and then measure the food accurately. That way you'll get a true picture of what you are really eating.

The nutritional analysis of my diet also showed I was getting more than the recommended dietary allowance (RDA) of vitamins and minerals, so I do not normally take supplements, not even a daily multivitamin, anymore. Also, my last cholesterol test indicated 154 total cholesterol, including 54 HDL (the good cholesterol), a very favorable ratio. If I have succeeded with my dietary goals, I believe there are two reasons: a healthy breakfast and Joanne Milkereit's refrigerator.

1. A HEALTHY BREAKFAST

You can think of a good breakfast as a fast start out of the blocks. Most mornings, I drink an 8-ounce glass of orange juice mixed with cranberry juice and eat a high-fiber, whole-grain breakfast cereal with fat-free milk, piled high with raisins, bananas, and whatever other fruits are in season: strawberries, raspberries, blueberries. In Florida, I found a specialty grocery store (Fresh Market) that offers dried cranberries, a treat to which

I have become addicted. A couple of times when we were out of milk, I substituted orange juice on my cereal. Yes, it sounds disgusting, but don't knock it until you've tried it.

I used to add two slices of toast spread with margarine or butter, and sometimes a soft-boiled egg, although as my mileage totals declined, I began to cut back on my calorie consumption to maintain a steady weight. Now, since protein needs increase with aging, Nancy Clark suggests I add eggs (or Greek yogurt or cottage cheese), given the lack of protein in my breakfast.

Sometimes on Sundays, between my long run and church, my wife and I will treat ourselves to a special breakfast with coffee cake (or pancakes, waffles, or French toast), bacon, and scrambled eggs with mozzarella cheese. Research suggests that if you are going to do any "fun" eating of high-fat foods, it is best to do it on days when you burn a lot of calories and can quickly metabolize those foods. This fits Clark's mantra that a diet can be 90 percent "quality foods" and 10 percent "stuff," if desired. (Nancy has been known to offer chocolate cake dispensations for important family events, such as birthdays.)

2. JOANNE MILKEREIT'S REFRIGERATOR

Let me tell you about Joanne Milkereit's refrigerator. Joanne Milkereit, RD, was the nutritionist at the Hyde Park Co-Op, an upscale grocery store near the University of Chicago, when we collaborated to write *Runner's Cookbook* back in 1979.

While we were working on the cookbook, Milkereit told me that all runners should tape the following words on their refrigerators: *Eat a wide variety of lightly processed foods.* Go back and reread that. Think about it. By *wide variety*, she means you sample all the food groups. Milkereit says: "When you eat 'lightly processed,' not only do you get all the vitamins and minerals but you get the fiber in plant foods." It is amazing that after all the nutritional research done in the past century, those words of advice remain valid.

What does Milkereit mean by *lightly processed*? Beware of foods that come wrapped in plastic or that you can buy at a fast-food restaurant—although restaurants have begun to offer such fare as low-fat burgers, carrot sticks, and nutritious salads. "Frankly," says Milkereit, "I feel we sometimes dump on fast-food restaurants too much. There are good choices in fast-food restaurants and bad choices in other restaurants."

Another food rule comes from Pete Pfitzinger, a 1984 and 1988 Olympic marathoner. He once told me, "I don't put anything in my mouth that's been invented in the last 25 years." That may be a bit extreme, Pete, but if you pay attention to these two messages—you eat primarily "real" foods; preferably, locally grown—you probably cannot go too wrong with your diet.

Fad diets offer little more than a trap for distance runners.

Judy Tillapaugh, RD, of Fort Wayne, Indiana, believes that although runners understand the value of carbo-loading before a marathon, they do not give equal attention to day-to-day meal plans. "Endurance athletes need to continually replace energy stores with a diet high in nutrient-dense carbohydrates, low in fat, and with enough protein to maintain muscle," says Tillapaugh. "Some weight-conscious runners don't eat enough." Clark agrees: "You can compete at your best only if you can train at your best. You can train at your best only if you fuel wisely and well on a day-to-day basis."

And you need to spread your calories throughout the day by snacking, choosing healthy fare such as fruit, graham crackers, yogurt, or whole-grain bagels. If you need 3,500 calories daily, you can't pack them into one or two meals. Athletes often neglect breakfast, then wonder why they are tired while running in the evening.

Fancy supplements, legal or illegal, cannot substitute for good nutrition. Excessive intake of vitamins is a waste of money and, in the case of fat-soluble vitamins (A, D, E, and K), raises a possible threat of long-term health problems. Dr. Applegate suggests taking a multivitamin that contains iron and zinc every other day as a minimum dosage. "Younger women need more iron than postmenopausal women," she says, "as do men who don't eat meat."

Eating a small 3-ounce portion of lean red meat two to four times a week can do a lot to make vitamin and mineral supplementation unnecessary; so can eating oily fish twice a week. I do both.

Can certain supplements improve performance? Apparently they can, judging from all the effort that goes into detecting their use by athletes competing at the Olympic level and in most professional sports. Drug use seems endemic in many sports, but in reality, probably only a relatively small percentage of athletes still try to steal an edge by using steroids or other performance-boosting drugs. Testing at major events and also outside competition is designed not only to catch cheaters for the benefit of drug-free athletes but also to prevent them from making mistakes that may shorten their life-spans.

Eat a wide variety of lightly processed foods.

I worry also about drug use by more ordinary athletes, those in the middle of the pack, who might be tempted to cut corners to set a PR or achieve a BQ. Nobody is testing this group, so who knows what negative behavior patterns exist?

LAST-MINUTE LOADING

Carbo-loading should not start or stop with the pasta dinner; scientists tell us it should continue throughout daily training routine and to the starting line to ensure maximum prerace nutrition. What you eat the day before the race fuels your muscles. What you eat the day of the race feeds the brain and tops off the muscles, too. W. Michael Sherman, PhD, an exercise scientist and sports nutrition expert from Ohio State University, tested trained cyclists pedaling indoors, feeding them 5 grams of carbohydrates per kilogram of body weight (2.25 g carb/pound) 3 hours before exercising. Both power and endurance increased when the athletes ate before exercising. (For a 165-pound cyclist, that would be about 1,500 calories from carbohydrate, the amount in twelve bagels or seven baked potatoes.) Dr. Sherman explains: "The cyclists were able to maintain a higher output for a longer period of time before fatiguing."

Other studies have shown improved performance 4 hours after eating. "We can safely say that if you have a carbohydrate feeding 3 to 4 hours before a marathon, you can enhance performance," says Dr. Sherman.

Admittedly, marathoners do not tolerate solids in their stomachs as well as cyclists do. Dr. Sherman suggests that runners either delay eating their prerace pasta until late evening or rise early for a carbohydrate-rich breakfast, such as oatmeal with raisins, or toast with honey, plus a glass of orange juice—foods that are tried-and-true, that you have eaten before your long training runs. If the fear of undesired pit stops requires you to abstain from fuel shortly before the event, sports nutritionist Nancy Clark suggests eating your breakfast the night before the marathon, right before you go to bed. This food will help maintain a normal blood sugar level, as well as your ability to think clearly and enjoy the race.

Liquid meals featuring high-carbohydrate drinks may work best for races near dawn. Dr. Sherman warns, however, that runners should try this first in practice or before minor races. You may find that if you consume too much immediately before the race, you waste time standing in portable-toilet lines both before and during the marathon.

Actually, practice may help you adjust to a different type of prerace nutrition that you may not have thought possible, including solid food an hour before the race. "You can train your body to do almost anything," says Tillapaugh, who says her favorite snack before races is a bagel or low-fat crackers.

"The main thing is not to do anything out of the ordinary," says Ed Eyestone, a 1988 and 1992 Olympic marathoner. "Yet you have to be flexible enough to go with the flow and eat what's available. If you're programmed to eat pancakes precisely 7 hours before a marathon, you may be disappointed."

Experience has taught me that eating as close as 3 hours before a race gives my stomach sufficient time to digest the food and allows me to clear my intestines without the fear of having to duck into the bushes at the 5-mile mark. Closer to race time than that, however, and I'm asking for trouble. Timing can be a problem when running a race like the Honolulu Marathon, with its predawn start. But I have gotten up as early as 2:30 a.m. to eat breakfast before that race, and I notice I am not always alone in the hotel coffee shop.

I will order orange juice, toast or maybe a Danish, and/or some applesauce, along with a single cup of coffee to help clear my bowels. We now know that caffeine, once thought to have a diuretic effect, does not contribute to dehydration. But it does contribute to enhanced stamina and endurance.

If you are running an international race—and I have run marathons in Berlin, Athens, Rome, Melbourne, and other major cities—you may not be able to get a typical American breakfast, but the continental breakfast of coffee and rolls (with or without jelly) works quite well.

If the coffee shop does not open early enough, those snacks in the suitcase may come in handy. I am even less fussy. Practically every hotel has a soft drink machine on each floor, and frequently a can of pop is my last meal before a morning marathon.

I stop drinking 2 hours before the race, as it takes approximately that long for liquids to migrate from your mouth to your bladder. Another cup or two just before the start will help you tank up for the race, and this liquid will most likely be used before it reaches your bladder. If you drink too much in that 2-hour period, however, you may find yourself worrying about how you will relieve yourself several miles into the race.

Following his bronze medal performance at the 1991 World Championships, Steve Spence told *Runner's World* that he drank so much that he had to urinate three times during the race without breaking stride. Personally, I prefer to avoid that. Experience teaches you how.

NO TREATS?

Does following a good sports diet mean no treats? My measured intake of 16 percent of calories from simple carbohydrates might be considered high for "healthy" people but not necessarily for a competitive runner. "Athletes are told to avoid junk foods," says Dr. Grandjean, "but the reality is that if you are eating 4,000 calories a day, once you have taken in those first 2,000 calories—assuming you've done a reasonably intelligent job of selecting foods—you've probably obtained all the nutrients you need. You don't need to worry about vitamins and minerals because you've already supplied your needs. You can afford foods high in sugar, so-called empty calories, because you just need energy. Your problem sometimes is finding enough time to eat." And yet, fueling your body with primarily premium nutrition is an investment in optimal health, Clark reminds us.

"You can compete at your best only if you can train at your best."

Sports nutrition thus comes down to time management.

The importance of general daily nutrition—as opposed to prerace nutrition—is that you need adequate energy for training and adequate nutrients to stay healthy plus heal the micro-injuries that occur during hard training sessions. And unlike the general population, you may need to eat more to help maintain your weight. If you are a 150-pound person running 30 miles a week to prepare for a marathon, you need approximately 3,000 calories a week more than if not running—assuming you maintain the same level of activity throughout the rest of your day. All too often, runners compensate for their "morning workout" by conserving energy the rest of the day. That is why some runners are unable to eat as much as they would like to be able to consume (without gaining weight, that is).

Most of those calories burned during exercise should be replaced with grains, fruits, and vegetables. Since those types of carbohydrates are bulkier than sugar, fats, or protein, the sheer volume of food that high-mileage runners must eat can become a problem.

Dr. Grandjean says that among the athletes she advises, distance runners are most knowledgeable about nutrition because their energy needs are so high. And those most talented, the ones already on top, often have the best nutrition. Fred Brouns of the Nutrition Research Center at the University of Limburg in the Netherlands studied cyclists competing in the Tour de France, both in the laboratory and during the race. He discovered that cyclists who finished near the front were those who were most successful at managing their diet. "Endurance athletes must pay close attention to food intake if they expect to keep energy levels high," says Brouns.

In the Tour de France, cyclists frequently burn 5,000 calories a day! There is no way these competitors can ride 5 or 6 hours a day and have time to eat that much, so they take many of their calories in liquid form while riding. Although most runners do not have anywhere near the energy requirements of a Tour cyclist, some high-mileage runners like to use high-carbohydrate drinks as a dietary supplement.

"If you have a carbohydrate feeding 3 to 4 hours before a marathon, you can enhance performance."

Nancy Ditz, the top U.S. finisher at the 1987 World Championships and 1988 Olympic marathons, took an intelligent approach to diet. Between those two marathons, Ditz decided she wanted to leave nothing to chance when it came to race preparation. Following the suggestion of her coach, Rod Dixon (the 1983 New York City Marathon champion and Olympic runner from New Zealand), she sought nutritional advice from Jerry Attaway, an assistant coach with the San Francisco 49ers. Attaway managed the team's strength training, rehabilitation, and diet programs. He determined that based on Ditz's energy expenditure while training 100 miles a week, she needed a higher percentage of carbohydrates than she was getting.

"Even though I was eating a pretty good diet, my carbohydrate intake still wasn't enough," Ditz recalls. She started using Exceed, a high-carbohydrate drink. (Such drinks are most effective when consumed immediately after exercise, when they can be most quickly absorbed.) Her calcium intake needed to be higher, so she also started drinking buttermilk with meals. Today's runners simply enjoy a tall glass of low-fat chocolate milk to help them get the carbs, protein, and calcium they desire.

Ditz feared Attaway might ask her to cut out one of her favorite treats—cinnamon rolls at breakfast—but instead he eliminated mayonnaise on her sandwich at lunch. "That was a minor behavioral change for a major change in my ratio of fat to carbohydrate," she says. (In 2 tablespoons of mayonnaise, you get 200 calories that are 100 percent fat!)

Attaway identified foods that did the most damage to Ditz's diet, then asked, "Which do you really like?" He let her keep those, then eliminated the rest.

Ideally, long-distance runners interested in maximizing their performance in the marathon should find a knowledgeable sports dietitian to teach them how to eat. If I had to offer a single piece of dietary advice to every person who reads this book—regardless of whether you have Olympic aspirations—it would be to consult a dietitian. That RD behind the name of a sports consultant can be the major portal to better performance and good health. The referral network of the Academy of Nutrition and Dietetics (eatright.org) can help you find a sports nutritionist. For a board-certified specialist in sports dietetics (CSSD), use the referral network at scandpg.org. Have that dietitian analyze your diet and recommend when, why, and what to eat for optimal performance.

DIET CHOICES

Do runners believe me when I tell them to follow a diet that is high in carbohydrates? More to the point, do they believe Nancy Clark, RD, author of the bestselling *Nancy Clark's Sports Nutrition Guide*? I asked Nancy to join me in conducting a survey on Twitter. We asked her Twitter followers what diet they use to fuel their workouts: Plants? Meats? Fats? Here is what we learned.

Diet choice	Percentage
High-carb, plant-based	42%
High-fat, as in the keto diet	4%
High-protein, as in the paleo diet	7%
None of the above	47%

Encouraging was the fact that neither the keto diet nor the paleo diet gained much traction among Clark's followers. Carbs ruled the day—except nearly half of those who took the survey admitted they followed no particular diet! Obviously, we have some educating to do.

The advice offered in this chapter should help you get to the starting line ready to perform. In a later chapter I will offer more nutritional information on what to drink and eat between that starting line and the finish line at mile 26.2.

19

The Perfect Pace

Steady as You Go

One year at the Chicago Marathon, Greg Castady of Homewood, Illinois, ran what he considered the near-perfect race at a near-perfect pace. He covered the first half in 1:25:28 and the second half in 1:25:21—only a 7-second spread en route to 2:50:49. Still, Castady was not entirely satisfied, saying, "I crossed the finish line thinking that I should have picked it up sooner because I felt I had more in the tank."

Four years later, also at Chicago, Castady ran a more aggressive race, running the first half in 1:20:19. Then, as winds picked up in the closing miles, he faded, covering the second half in 1:28:03. Although his time of 2:48:03 set a new personal record by nearly 3 minutes, he wondered what he might have accomplished if he had paced the race better. "I suppose that when I hit that mythical 'perfect race,' I can retire from marathon running," he said.

Finally, five years after that, Castady returned to Chicago one more time and ran that perfect race, hitting "negative splits," going out in 1:17:49 and finishing in 1:17:16 for a PR of 2:35:05. He was a much fitter runner but also a much smarter runner—at least in the area of pacing.

Castady, however, said he was not yet ready to retire: "I still have a few marathons left in me."

We all seek the perfect race, in which we achieve the perfect pace, crossing the finish line with no energy left—running on fumes, so to speak—aware that we could not have run one second faster, gone one step farther. *"Thanks for hanging the medal around my neck, but I am about ready to fall on my face."* Perfect pace is not always easy to accomplish, but dreaming the impossible dream is part of what sends us to the starting line time and time again.

"The key," suggests Liz Reichman of San Antonio, "seems to be estimating your fitness accurately. That allows you to run even splits. Overestimate your ability and you struggle the second half."

But how do you estimate fitness and pick the pace that is right for you? How do you determine a reasonable finishing time? These are vexing questions, not only for experienced runners but particularly for first-time marathoners—new runners with no background of past performances for guidance.

We all seek the perfect race, in which we achieve the perfect pace.

If you never have run a marathon race before, how can you have a "race pace"? This troubles newcomers when they launch themselves into the unpredictable waters of our sport.

Unless you have at least some idea of the time you are capable of recording in a marathon, you will not know how fast to run each of the 26 miles en route to that time. Run too slowly at the start and you may find yourself too fresh at the end and with a slower finishing time than you had anticipated. That is okay if you are a first-timer intent only on finishing, but not if you are a seasoned runner like Greg Castady hoping to improve.

The other side of the competitive coin can be more of a problem. Start too quickly and you may find yourself struggling by the 20-mile mark, that mythical point that some runners refer to as the wall. Twenty miles is about the point on the course where many marathoners start coming unglued as they fall off their carefully planned paces. The bear drops onto their shoulders. They get a case of the "riggies" as rigor mortis sets in. Suddenly, running becomes much, much more difficult, and they may be forced to slow down or walk or even stop. Running an even pace is the best way to avoid hitting the wall, or so goes the conventional wisdom.

FINDING YOUR PACE

Achieving that perfect pace, however, is not always easy. Here are three ways to determine your marathon pace.

1. WORKOUTS

If you chart your times during workouts—speed workouts as well as your long runs—you probably have an idea of how fast you can run. But that's only an approximate idea. It is not always easy to interpolate workout data in order to be able to predict performance. I hate being the harbinger of bad news, but just because you can run an 8:00 pace for 20 miles, there is no guarantee that you can run that same pace for 26 miles 385 yards. You may be forced to run slower, or—if you paid attention to what I said earlier and ran your long runs at a comfortable pace—you may actually be able to run faster!

Predicting performance from workouts probably works better for experienced runners than for first-timers, particularly experienced runners who record their training in logs or a diary. These vets often have a "feel" for fitness, based on previous workouts leading up to previous marathons. If you are running significantly faster on your easy runs, as well as on your hard runs, and perhaps logging more miles as well, that suggests you may have achieved a higher fitness level that may result in a faster time.

2. SHORT-DISTANCE RACES

A somewhat more accurate gauge of potential are your times in preliminary races at popular submarathon distances, from 5K through the half
marathon. First-timers can get at least a hint of their potential and build
confidence by running some races during their marathon buildup. Experienced runners can confirm whether what seems to be improved fitness
is real or imagined. But this can work in reverse, too. If your fitness has
declined since your last marathon, you will want to know so you can set a
somewhat lower goal. Fortunately, various performance charts allow you
to estimate how fast you can run a marathon. In my various marathon
training programs lasting 18 weeks, I usually suggest a test race around
Week 8 or 9 to help runners (new and old) with their race predictions.

3. PREVIOUS MARATHONS

A better gauge, at least for experienced runners, is how fast you ran in previous marathons. If you ran 4:10 in your last marathon and have increased
your level of training, you might have a reasonable chance of breaking 4
hours your next time out. Notice the qualifying "might." There is never
any guarantee. Difficulty of the course, weather conditions, an unex-
pected injury, that cold you had last week—anything could thwart your
ambitions.

The more marathons you run, the easier it becomes to predict performance based on experience. If you are a first-timer, the best strategy is
to be conservative in your predictions, knowing that the most important
goal is crossing the finish line, regardless of time. Think carefully about
how fast you want to run your first marathon. Then add a half hour to
that time! If you reach 13 miles and realize you are woefully underpaced,
curse me loudly and speed up, knowing you certainly should be able to
run your second marathon faster.

Although most runners will tell you that the best strategy is to run
even pace or negative splits (second half faster than the first), most of
those responding to an Internet poll I conducted admitted that in their

PR races, they had slowed in the second half—a third of them by as much as 3 to 5 minutes.

Inevitably, predicting pace becomes a guessing game on the part of every runner. In some respects, the unpredictability of the marathon is what makes it such an exciting adventure. If you have run three or four previous marathons, you can afford to take a risk by going out too fast and hoping to hang on. Nevertheless, runners can obtain some help from scientists and mathematicians in trying to determine just how fast they might run in a marathon, be it their first marathon or one in which they hope to set a PR.

PREDICTING PERFORMANCE

With the increased interest in fitness sports during the past several decades, there has been a simultaneous rise in the number of laboratories that are dedicated to measuring human performance. Scientists continue to explore why some athletes outperform others.

The most common measuring device found in any running-oriented human performance laboratory is the treadmill, a moving belt on which you run in place while exercise scientists take various measurements. The most common measurement is VO_2 max, the volume of oxygen a person can consume during exercise. This relates both to the heart's capacity to pump oxygen-rich blood to the muscles and to how efficiently the muscles extract and use that oxygen.

Start too quickly and you may find yourself struggling by the 20-mile mark.

If you know your max, you can come close to estimating your marathon time. Jack Daniels, PhD, a former coach at the State University of New York, pioneered the use of VO_2 max to predict performance. In fact, I borrowed Dr. Daniels's charts for the first three editions of this book to help runners predict how fast they might run a marathon based on their lab scores or race times for distances 1 mile and longer.

The Daniels tables still serve as a handy reference, but marathoners seeking to predict times are more likely nowadays to use the Internet. I often refer runners to a calculator on the website mcmillanrunning.com, the work of Greg McMillan, a national champion marathoner from Mill Valley, California. McMillan's Running Calculator operates with supreme simplicity. Input your running time at any one of 28 distances, from 100 meters to 100 miles, and the calculator quickly estimates your potential time at all the other distances.

IS PREDICTION POSSIBLE?

How well do prediction calculators work? Very well—on average. Whether designed by Jack Daniels, Greg McMillan, *Runner's World*, or others, calculators offer a reasonable estimate to aid most runners in predicting marathon performance. But invariably in calculations involving humans with differing abilities, not everybody fits comfortably into the bell curve. Some runners are born sprinters; others are born marathoners.

The world record for 200 meters, as of this writing, is held by Jamaica's Usain Bolt, who ran 19.19 at the 2009 World Track and Field Championships. The McMillan calculator does not convert from hundredths of a second, but a 19-second 200 predicts a mind-shattering 1:48:53 for the marathon! That is nearly 13 minutes faster than the 2:01:39 that Eliud Kipchoge of Kenya ran at the 2018 Berlin Marathon.

In truth, sprinters succeed because they possess muscular physiques and a preponderance of fast-twitch muscles. Marathoners succeed because they are lean and light and have a preponderance of slow-twitch muscles. Ordinary runners who do not match these extraordinary athletes sit somewhere in between, probably closer to the top of the bell curve. Everybody has a perfect distance, or range of distances, at which they perform best. If you fail to match a calculator's prediction, it may not be the fault of your training. In the meantime, take with a grain of salt how fast any coach or computer suggests you can run a marathon. Using McMillan's Running Calculator, here are some common conversions from 5K times to the half and full marathon.

5K	Half Marathon	Marathon
15:00	1:09:20	2:26:14
20:00	1:32:27	3:14:58
25:00	1:55:34	4:03:44
30:00	2:18:40	4:52:28
35:00	2:41:47	5:41:12
40:00	3:04:54	6:29:57
45:00	3:28:01	7:18:42

For more precise calculations, visit mcmillanrunning.com.

Converting potential into performance provides runners with their biggest challenge. Using a 5K time to predict a marathon time does not work as well as using the time from a longer race, such as a half marathon—or best, a 25K, and there are several good races at that distance. But even interpolating half to full can be tricky. Some runners have more fast-twitch muscles than slow-twitch. They are born sprinters who may struggle in an event that requires more endurance than speed for success. The reverse is that runners with more endurance than speed, and who do not train to maximize what little speed they possess, also may find it difficult when prediction meets reality at the 20-mile mark.

Achieving success as a long-distance runner, then, remains as much an art as a science. You need to apply both art and science if you expect to succeed.

Pick a realistic goal. For first-timers, it should be a conservative goal. Indeed, a large part of why many runners hit the wall at 20 miles may be the result of their not having accurately estimated their own abilities. If you train properly and pick a reasonable pace, there should be no wall.

PACING TEAMS

Once you obtain an estimate of your finishing time, you can determine the best means of achieving that time. Many major marathons now offer pacing teams to aid runners in achieving their goals, whether those goals are to run a fast time or, most simply, to finish. Pacing teams usually are led by experienced runners, who promise to run an even pace to help other runners achieve a specific goal time. If the goal is a 4:30 marathon, the pace team leader will attempt to run a steady 10:18 pace, team members tucked behind like goslings behind a goose, knowing that if they stick near that leader, they will achieve their goals. Even if they drop off that pace, which often happens, they are reasonably certain of running at least a good time or of finishing. I have led pacing teams at Chicago, Disney World, and Honolulu, and it is a lot of fun for both the leader and the followers.

Achieving success as a long-distance runner remains as much an art as a science.

Credit for developing the pacing team concept goes to the former *Runner's World* editor and Boston Marathon champ Amby Burfoot, although I provided some of the spark because of an article, "Fast Train to Boston," that I wrote for the July 1995 issue of *Runner's World*. It was during a period when the goal of many runners was to qualify for the 100th running of the Boston Marathon, a landmark event that eventually attracted a record 35,868 finishers.

Using data provided by ninety-one different marathons and convening an expert panel of five members of the Road Runners Club of America, I picked the ten fall marathons whose courses seemed most likely to yield a qualifying time. Top of the heap was the St. George Marathon in Utah, whose mostly downhill course dropped 2,600 feet from mountains to the valley. (For a list of the ten top marathons that provide the most Boston qualifiers, see page 313.)

With that as inspiration, Burfoot gathered a group of *Runner's World* editors, most of them experienced marathoners, and traveled to St. George to help runners entered in that year's race qualify for Boston. They were enormously successful, with 1,030 of the 3,207 finishing runners—nearly a third of the field—qualifying for the 100th Boston Marathon.

Thus began the concept of *Runner's World* pacing teams, and in succeeding years, the magazine's editors traveled to Dallas, Chicago, Orlando (Disney World), Honolulu, Tucson, and Portland to pace runners. I missed the first two team efforts, but when Burfoot and crew arrived in Chicago, where I served as training consultant, I told race director Carey Pinkowski that we were going to steal their pace team idea the following year.

And we did, perfecting the concept because Chicago had more available volunteer leaders than *Runner's World* had editors. And the pacing teams kept getting bigger and better. Today, many major marathons provide pacing teams to help runners achieve their goals. The magazine eventually abandoned the pacing business, happy to have provided the spark that has helped so many marathoners to finish-line success. (To determine whether your marathon of choice offers pacing teams, simply check the race website.)

The pacing team operation at Chicago and other marathons works simply. At the expo before the marathon, runners stop by the pacing team booth to register to run and talk to leaders about their race strategies for the next day. Though some leaders run through aid stations, most in Chicago follow my advice and walk as they drink. Or they may employ other strategies that you need to know in advance. Registered runners receive numbers—such as 4:30 or 5:30—to pin to their backs, identifying them as members of that pacing team. "It helps keep everybody together in crowded fields," says Dennis Linehan, who has led pacing teams at numerous marathons. "It's easy to get separated when you pass through an aid station. The numbers on the back help lost runners regain contact."

The morning of the race, leaders meet early and grab large signs identifying their times. The leaders march out to the starting grid and position themselves on the right side of the grid so runners can easily find them. They also wear identical uniforms and caps. Once across the line, most set aside the large signs but continue to carry smaller numbered signs, sometimes for the entire race.

Maintaining the same pace for 26 miles is not easy, and as the race continues, invariably some people lose contact, then more, then more and more. As a pace team leader, I have noticed that almost everybody can handle the pace through 10 miles and into the half marathon. They converse with one another and wave back at spectators. But beyond the half marathon point, people start taking reality checks related to pace. One by one, they start slipping back. By 20 miles, usually the team is down to a small but tightly focused group that generally sticks together to hug one another in the finish chute.

If you're not planning to attach yourself to a pacing team, here are some strategies for picking your own pace and achieving your goals.

- Choose a realistic goal.
- Carry your pacing schedule with you so you can figure out how close you are to pace at every point in the race.
- Believe in your pace chart: Check each mile, making no changes in the first 20 miles (no matter how "good" you feel).
- Be prepared to make the necessary adjustments if the course is especially hilly.
- Meet intermediate time goals. This gives you confidence and causes the miles to pass faster.
- At mile 20, if you feel good, go for it; if not, hang in there.

One caveat concerning any pacing plan: Most pacing charts are designed under the assumption that the course is flat, with zero wind. If the course is hilly or the weather windy, you may need to make adjustments. A tailwind will make you run faster, sometimes as much as several minutes over the course of 26 miles. This certainly was proved true at the 2011 Boston Marathon, when on a day with a stiff wind at his back, Kenya's Geoffrey Mutai ran 2:03:02, 57 seconds faster than the listed world record. Because Boston's point-to-point and downhill course is considered to be "aided" under International Association of Athletic Federations standards, Mutai could be credited only with having run a "world best," not a world record.

> **At mile 20, if you feel good, go for it.**

On a loop course, where the wind may hit you from different directions at different times, you may need to make mental adjustments at midrace to stay on pace. Temperature can also affect pace. When race temperatures rise or fall much above or below your comfort level, you may need to throw your pace table away.

A pace table can be a trap, a series of numbers that can lure you into too fast a pace for your capabilities on any one day. The best pace-setting device becomes your own mind. Experienced runners eventually know when to slow down and when to speed up. Of course, it may take them more than a few marathons, and there always remains room for improvement. That is part of the fascination of running 26 miles 385 yards and doing it more than one time.

FINDING THE RIGHT PACE

Curious as to how most runners determined the pace they hoped to run in a marathon, I did a survey offering four possible choices. Interestingly, more than half of the runners claimed to pick their pace depending on how they felt in workouts, although it would

(continued)

seem that this strategy may not work for first-timers. The best approach might be to use workouts to determine your fitness, but use a prediction chart to determine whether you are right and, finally, at the race join a pacing team so you don't have to worry about your pace.

Pacing strategy	Percentage who use that strategy
How I feel in workouts	54%
Prediction charts	19%
Pace teams in race	8%
Don't worry about pace	19%

20

Race Day Logistics

The Big Day Has Come.
Are You Ready?

After 18 weeks or more of training—after the mileage buildup, the long runs, the taper, the carbo-loading, after your having reread this book three times—what can you expect once you arrive at the race site and head toward the starting line? Most veterans usually follow a well-rehearsed routine that makes their marathons easy (well, easier than they might otherwise be). Here are some suggestions that just might make race day easier for you.

Your "final" preparation begins just before you leave home, when you pack your bag. In this case, you need to heed the advice of one doctor: the late George Sheehan, MD, who for several decades wrote a monthly column for *Runner's World* that focused as much on philosophy as physiology. Dr. Sheehan never left home without his runner's suitcase, a bag in the trunk of his car packed with gear in case he stopped somewhere and wanted to run. Dr. Sheehan once wrote about the bag—then forgot it the next time he left for a 10-mile race in New York City's Van Cortlandt Park.

"I had to borrow shoes, shorts, and a shirt," Dr. Sheehan recalled. "I was completely outfitted by other runners, who fortunately hadn't forgotten their bags."

Before packing, consider the advice of Michigan's Doug Kurtis, who in addition to having won the Detroit Marathon a half-dozen times has also broken 3 hours two hundred times. Kurtis instructs: "Break everything in before you race: socks, shorts, singlet, shoes." Kurtis recommends running one or two workouts in your racing gear to make certain everything fits and there are no problem areas, such as an imperfection inside a shoe that could cause a blister. That may not bother you in a 5K, but it can draw blood and bring you to a halt in a marathon. "One good way to work out the bugs and test your equipment is to enter shorter races before the marathon," suggests Kurtis.

> **"Break everything in before you race."**

My general recommendation is to buy new shoes 3 to 6 weeks before the marathon so you have time to test them and get a different pair if the first pair causes problems. But I run in lightweight racing flats, whereas most runners prefer the extra protection offered by their everyday training shoes. Some first-timers own only a single pair and need to change if their shoes have too many miles on them.

As expected, different runners admit to different mileages. "I prefer racing in new shoes," says Cindy Southgate of Kanata, Ontario, "but invariably, I can't afford them at the right time or I'm too scared to shift too close to the race. I usually run marathons with about 200 miles on my shoes." In an Internet survey I conducted, more than half the participants admitted to wearing shoes with more than 100 miles on them for their marathons.

MILEAGE CHECK

Veteran runners usually have multiple pairs of shoes, including one pair that they reserve for races at various distances from the 5K to the half marathon, and often for fast workouts. Before important marathons, however, we head to the local specialty running shop to buy a new pair of racing flats, knowing that our shoes need to be shiny clean to guarantee that PR or BQ. But, following Doug Kurtis's advice, we do not want to race in shoes right out of the box. See in the following chart what percentage chose that option: only a handful of runners out of 660 respondents to the survey.

How many miles should we run in our new racing flats before using them in a marathon? I asked that question online and received these answers.

Miles on shoes before racing	Percentage
0 miles	1%
20 miles	18%
50 miles	28%
100 miles or more	53%

But not Ed Brickell of Dallas: "For my last several marathons, I ran with pairs right out of the box—although of a model I had trained with extensively."

David Harrison of Clitheroe, England, buys a new pair of shoes 6 weeks out. "I start using them for shorter distances," he says, "then do my last 20-miler in them. If something is going to rub, I want to know about it." The more you know about the shoes on your feet, the less chance a blister will halt you midstride.

A RUNNER'S BAG

Back to George Sheehan's bag: Running clothes and shoes are only the minimum essentials, whether you are heading for a workout or a race. Smart runners cram their bags with numerous other items. Here are some items you might want to include in your runner's suitcase, not only for the marathon, but for other road races.

The right shoes. The most essential item, as discussed earlier. But what about a second pair? Many runners (myself included) like to take training shoes for warming up or riding the bus to the start, then shift to a lighter pair of racing flats before heading to the starting line. On rainy days, you will want dry shoes for afterward. Also, make sure your pet pair of shoes makes it with you to the race. For security, you may want to pack your racing shoes in your carry-on luggage. If the airline loses your bag, you can replace everything else, but not a well-broken-in pair of shoes. I have never forgotten or lost my running shoes, but one winter en route to a 30K cross-country ski race in Ottawa, the airline lost my bag containing skis, poles, and boots. A friend lent me replacement equipment, including boots two sizes too large, but it was not a very enjoyable race.

Shorts and singlet. Some people wear the cotton race T-shirt they have been given at the expo the day before, but this is not a very bright procedure to follow. Cotton retains moisture: bad for both cold and hot weather. I also prefer to test *everything*! Do the shorts fit? Will the singlet or T-shirt chafe? (A snug shirt or a brand-new, unwashed one might.) You will be most comfortable standing at the starting line if you wait until after warming up to change into a dry racing singlet. You can shed the shirt a mile or two into the race knowing that the race director will have the course swept of unwanted gear that will go to the homeless. (But do not throw the shirt joyously in the air, since it may hit or trip a runner behind you.) Pin your number on the night before the race, and check to make sure you have not pinned the front of your singlet to the back. (Yes, I have done that, and it is an irritation to repin a number while standing on the starting line.)

Safety pins. Most races provide safety pins, but sometimes only two, and sometimes they run out. If you are like me, you will want at least four to secure your number so it does not flap. A few races require two numbers. At Twin Cities, you wear a back number identifying your age group, a nice touch if you are cruising for an award. (I won $250 one year for winning the 60-to-64 division.) If you are running in a marathon that provides pacing teams, you will need four pins to secure the back number identifying your team. Pins also come in handy for other things, such as piercing blisters after the race (although podiatrists may not like my offering such advice, since you are supposed to use a sterilized pin). I usually take along four or more pins linked together and fastened to a snap on the outside of my bag or in my toilet kit.

Check the race website for vital information.

Instructions. It made sense in the first four editions of this book when I suggested that runners bring the race entry blank, but paper entry blanks hardly exist anymore. Everyone enters online. So check the race website for vital information, including directions. At most major marathons, where you stay overnight in a hotel, getting lost trying to find the starting line is hardly a problem. Like lemmings, we follow other runners, who have gotten out of bed earlier. But it is a smart move to have good directions to the lower-number 5K or 10K you are running as a test race to get ready for the marathon.

Once you pick up your race number, there may be further instructions in the goody bag. Are you certain of the time the bus leaves for the start and when the start is? The race may begin at 7:45 a.m. to accommodate TV coverage, not the more logical 8:00 you seem to remember because it is an even number. On race day, use the time between the warmup and the start to read, one last time, all the directions you have accumulated. You may learn about some vital detail that will help you in the race, such as the location of aid stations or portable toilets.

Gloves and a cap. If the day is cold, you will want these extra items. Whether or not you wear them during the race, gloves and a cap can help you stay warm before and after. If you start a marathon in the morning cold but get too warm by midrace, you can always toss your gloves—or tuck them in the waistband of your shorts. A billed cap in summer will keep the sun off your face. This is a necessity to avoid sunburn that might lead to skin cancer later in life. Caps come in handy to keep rain or—I hate to mention this—snow off your face. As with other race gear, test each item for comfort during practice. Until companies began to provide high-tech caps for running, I wore a torn and battered cotton cap so formless and ugly that I would not want to be seen in it anywhere but on the starting line of a marathon. Painter's caps also were very popular among the previous era's runners. Another old road runner trick was to knot a white handkerchief at its four corners to wear on the head. I have not seen that for a while.

Varied-weight clothing. Do not assume the weather will be warm if the month is July or cold if it is January. If a freak cold wave or heat wave hits, can you cope with it? The Boston Marathon in April is notorious for unpredictable weather. I wear shorts and a regular race singlet if the temperature is going to be in the mid-40s. If it is much colder, I will don Lycra tights and a long-sleeved shirt—a big improvement over the heavy cotton turtleneck I had to wear for warmth in the cold and rainy 1964 Boston Marathon when I set my PR. (Yes, I could have run at least 10 minutes faster if I'd been properly clad.) Along with your gloves and hat, pack a headband to cover your ears on really cold days.

Have you forgotten anything?

Throwaway clothing. In large races, where you may need to stand on the starting line for a long time, it is important to stay warm. If you cannot hand your discarded warmup gear to a friend at the last minute, take throwaway clothes that you will not mind having donated to the Salvation Army or Goodwill when you leave them behind. Garbage bags with armholes cut in them protect against the wind and wet but do not hold much warmth. Most major marathons arrange to both collect your bag before the race and deliver it to you after, but you may need to strip off your warmup suit and tuck it into your bag a half hour or more before the start. Also, be sure to determine before race day what kind of bag-checking system will be in place. At smaller races there may be no system, meaning you are responsible for your own gear. Particularly in crowded fields, you may need to stand a long time on the starting grid. Fortunately, most marathons today are so well organized that they start precisely on time.

One important point for your benefit and for the benefit of runners behind you on the starting grid: Do not—repeat, do not—remove and hurl items of clothing into the air when the gun goes off. It looks good on TV, but it means that others behind you will have to step over your discarded items. Discard your clothing on the curb or hand it to a spectator along the course, even if it means carrying the clothing for a while until you can move to one side. If you trip over a sweatshirt dropped on the course, it was probably dropped by some idiot who failed to read this book.

SOME FURTHER SMALL ITEMS

Here are some other items you could easily forget as you focus on the task at hand. But including them in your race day planning will make your experience more enjoyable.

Fluids and food. Need a final prerace drink, either water or your favorite sports drink? It is easier to sip from a bottle you brought along than to go searching for fluids. Gels are handy for midrace carb-reloading. If you do not have shorts with pockets, you will be happy I told you to pack extra safety pins so you can attach the gel packets to your singlet. Although most marathons will have bananas, yogurt, and other food items waiting for you after you clear the finish chute, if you finish too far back, you may find they have run out. Or—and this has happened to me more than once—you may stagger head down through the finish area

(continued)

and retrieve your bag before realizing you missed the food tables entirely and need to go back. (Traffic coming out may make returning impossible to accomplish.)

Combination lock. This comes in handy if there is a dressing room where you can stow your gear in a locker, although access to lockers is more common at track meets than at marathons. Many races today are so large that runners come dressed to run.

Postrace clothing. Once you finish, you will want to change into dry clothing, including socks. Make sure you pack a towel so you can dry off. You will want to look and feel your best hanging around and chatting with other runners. This is important for workouts, too. I do most of my running from home, but when I climb in the car to drive to some scenic area, such as Indiana Dunes State Park, I bring a change of clothes, whether it is a hot or cold day. It's easy to get chilled driving home while wearing a shirt soaked with sweat.

Plastic bag. Plastic bags come in handy after the race to isolate your wet and sweaty gear from the rest of your clothing. A separate plastic bag for grimy shoes is also useful if your marathon is on trails rather than on pavement.

Miscellaneous. Today's electronic devices contain so much memory, from split times to maps of the course just run, that the advice I offered in earlier editions suggesting you bring a pen and notebook to record your finishing time may be obsolete. But bring them anyway. Maybe at the 18-mile mark, you'll meet a good-looking gal or guy whose phone number you will want to jot down. Yes, that happened to a friend of mine running the Honolulu Marathon and they spent the next several days together seeing the islands.

Checklist. Have you forgotten anything? You won't know unless you also have a checklist of all the necessary items. Experience eventually will guide you. When you determine what items work best in your runner's bag, make a personalized checklist similar to the one in the Race Day Checklist on page 261.

Money. Of course, you will need money the day of the race for your entry fee if you have not preregistered. (Race day registration is more common for smaller and shorter races than for marathons.) Cash also comes in handy after the race if a vendor is sell-ing ice cream—or so you can take the subway home if you locked your keys in the car. Put a few extra dollars and some change in the bag that gets transported to the finish line just in case you need it. Is there a chance you might drop out? Tuck a $20 bill in your shorts pocket so you can grab a taxi. It is not a wise idea to place your wallet or valuable items in the bags you check. Most races warn runners against this prac-tice. If you do place a cellphone in your bag (and I am not advising that), turn it off so it will not start ringing in the baggage area.

> **Becoming toilet trained is a necessity.**

Extra little essentials. Pack these in a smaller bag: anti-chafing lubri-cants, adhesive bandages, tape, sunscreen, aspirin, and other medication. Sure, you may be able to buy some or all of these items at the race expo, but do not leave any essential items home based on that assumption. You do not want to have to be told, "Sorry, we're all sold out."

THE MORNING OF THE RACE

For 5K or 10K races, I do not mind rising early and driving an hour or two to run, and most runners feel the same. Not only do I want to avoid the extra expense of a hotel and meals away from home, but an overnight stay converts a fun race into an expedition requiring planning and com-mitment. Sometimes I like to just go, run, and head home, not waiting for the awards ceremony (which may take forever) unless I have won an age-group prize and don't want to have my name read out loud, which causes everybody to look around and wonder where I went.

But a marathon does require commitment, so I prefer to stay over-night before the race. I have run the Sunburst Marathon in South Bend,

Indiana, on several occasions. Even though South Bend is only 45 minutes from my home in Long Beach, I checked into a hotel the night before the event to avoid having to drive even that far on race morning and to allow myself an extra hour's sleep before a 6:00 a.m. start. And for major marathons, particularly if you are bringing your family, you may want to arrive 2 or 3 days early to do some sightseeing and partake in numerous race activities. Did you really sign up for the Disney World Marathon thinking that you could avoid the theme parks? Your kids didn't think so.

Even if it costs a little more, I prefer to stay as close as possible to the race's start and/or finish. Usually race directors select their headquarters hotel with this in mind, negotiating blocks of rooms at discounts for runners who reserve early. Having a hotel near the start will allow you to wait in your room until the last minute before heading downstairs. Access to a last-minute restroom where the floor is tile (in your hotel room) rather than plastic (in an outdoor portable toilet) is an important perk. Right after finishing the race, you can return to your room for a cleansing shower. For point-to-point marathons, most runners stay near the finish line so they can head to their rooms quickly after finishing. But make your hotel reservations early, because the most desirable hotels at big-city marathons often fill up fast, sometimes a year in advance. Also, once the reduced-rate rooms disappear, the prices can go up—way up!

Boston has a devilishly difficult course.

You do not want to sleep through the start or oversleep and have to rush your final preparations. This is particularly true at marathons that begin very early in the morning, such as Honolulu with its 5:00 a.m. start. Usually my internal body alarm wakes me up a few minutes before the actual alarm sounds (maybe I do not want to hear its jarring noise). Before important races I will set my wristwatch alarm, set the clock radio alarm, and even ask the front desk for a wake-up call. If you are a really heavy sleeper, have a friend at home call you on the phone and stay on the line until you have stumbled out of bed.

Your first assignment after rising is to complete your carbo-load by either going down to the hotel coffee shop or snacking on items brought with you for that purpose. My favorite prerace "meal" is usually orange juice, a Danish, and a cup of coffee 3 hours out. Two hours out, I might have something else to drink. But that will be my last food or drink before the start, because I do not want to have to use a toilet once the race begins. Two hours usually is enough to allow everything to settle. Energy bars also can provide an effective last-minute meal, but be sure you eat one that is mostly carbohydrate. Some bars contain extra protein, good for postmarathon recovery but not necessarily what you need before the race.

I often do a very short warmup at the hotel an hour or more before the start, for several reasons. First, going outside and testing the weather is more reliable than listening to weather reports on TV or the radio. Second, a short run usually loosens my bowels; I would rather use the toilet in my hotel room than stand in a long line for a portable toilet. A half mile or so of jogging and walking usually accomplishes this.

Becoming toilet trained is a necessity if you do not want to waste energy and time waiting to use a portable toilet. Ideally, you will have determined during your long runs in training what foods provide the least intestinal distress (not everybody can handle pasta), but prerace nerves may trick your system. If I am driving to the start, I sometimes arrive with a nearly empty gas tank so I will have an excuse to stop at a gas station and use the restroom. I am adept at locating toilets that I can visit during my warmup. Driving the final miles to the race, I keep my eyes open for a friendly fast-food restaurant close enough to jog to but far enough away so most of the other runners will not head for it. That is one advantage of being a high-mileage runner: You can outrun the competition to reach an uncrowded toilet.

For my early-morning warmup, I do not usually wear my racing gear. After visiting the john and changing, I gather any extra gear I need—including my runner's bag, packed the night before—and head for the start.

THE STARTING LINE

Each race has its own protocol requiring careful attention (and some experience—yours or that of friends) if you do not want to get to the starting line too early or too late. At the Boston Marathon, runners board buses in downtown Boston by 6:00 a.m. for transportation to where the race begins nearly 4 hours later. After arriving near the start, they spend the next hour or two milling around in the athletes' village outside the high school in suburban Hopkinton before being shooed to the starting line 30 to 60 minutes before the race begins. Weather can turn a good prerace experience into a bad one, so you need to learn each race's logistics to stay as warm and dry as possible.

At Boston and most other large races, the elite runners are supplied with transportation and a private dressing area near the start. It makes the final hour before the marathon much more comfortable, a necessity for runners seeking peak performance. Because race directors hope for fast times to please sponsors, they do what they can to make the prerace conditions comfortable for top competitors. But most race directors do a good job for the rest of us as well. Particularly during the fall marathon season, there is a lot of competition among race directors to make the runners comfortable so that they will return in subsequent years and provide the numbers the sponsors like. Fortunately, many race directors are marathoners (or former marathoners) themselves and remember the types of user-friendly practices that kept them comfortable and happy. During the year when I crammed seven marathons into 7 months to commemorate my 70th birthday, I was struck by how well organized each race was and how well the race directors provided the back of the pack with a reasonable amount of comfort.

Runners without the privilege of the elite dressing room need to organize themselves as much as possible on race day to minimize the hassle caused by being part of a forty-thousand-runner event. This requires planning. Often you learn how to cope with one specific marathon only by running it once and returning the following year better prepared. Or, if you are lucky, you attend the race with friends who were there the year before and can tell you what to expect. I usually warn runners doing the Boston Marathon for the first time not to expect a PR effort no matter how well trained they think they are. Boston has a devilishly difficult course that almost needs to be run once before you can logically expect to run a fast time. Everything around the course must be learned, too. I figure it took me three or four times before I figured the race out, and that was when there were only a few hundred in the field. Runners often post questions online to learn about marathons they have not yet run. This is called networking, and it works in marathoning as well as it does in business and social life.

Warming up is difficult—if not impossible—at large races because at the time when you normally might do some final strides or a bit of jogging, you often need to stay in place to secure your position on the starting grid. At the really big marathons, such as Honolulu or Disney World, runners are marched to the line well before the gun. It is the only way to handle the crowds of starters, but if you like to follow a particular warmup routine, as I do, this arrangement can wreak havoc with your preparation. The fortunate thing about marathons is that unless you are an elite runner planning a 4:30 first mile, you probably do not need as much warmup as you might for a 5K race, where you need to run fast from the gun. You may lose a minute or two with a slow start, but this may not be that important over the length of a marathon. If you are a first-timer, you probably will not warm up because you do not want to waste even the tiny amount of energy it requires to jog in place standing on the line. Experienced runners, however, often have different agendas. The inconvenience of crowds is one reason you may want to try a small, intimate marathon when you attempt a new PR.

At races where I planned to compete for first in my age group, I used to position myself as close to the starting line as I could without blocking faster runners. I am somewhat less competitive now and often line up at the absolute back of the pack at races such as the Gate River Run, a 15K race I run every year in Jacksonville, Florida, near our winter home. One advantage of my last-row lineup scheme is that once the gun sounds, I can use a portable toilet without having to wait in a long line. The only time this got me in trouble was at the Comrades Marathon in South Africa, when I emerged from the toilet after taking too long and realized that the last runners were several blocks ahead of me down the street. It took me several kilometers to regain contact, during which time a police car pulled beside me and the officer asked, "Are you in the race?"

Position on the starting grid is less critical today than it was several decades ago; in practically every major marathon, computer chips (which are sometimes embedded in your race number) are used to provide runners with an official time that recognizes when they cross the starting line, not when the gun sounds. Leading a pacing team at the Chicago Marathon one year, I held the 5:00 group back until the starting line was nearly clear of runners. This meant crossing the line 8 minutes late. Since those "lost minutes" would be subtracted from everybody's official time, it did not really matter when we started.

My team experienced no delays caused by runners around us and actually ran the first 2 miles somewhat faster than our planned pace. Several months later at the Disney World Marathon, where I led the 4:30 pacing team for *Runner's World*, it took only 4 minutes to cross the line, but we lost a minute a mile for the first 3 miles because of a narrower course. That was before Disney split its half marathon and marathon; they are now run on consecutive days and include the popular Dopey Challenge with a 5K, 10K, half marathon, and full marathon on 4 days. Every marathon is slightly different, so you need to approach each with a plan that is both flexible and well defined. Only by understanding race day logistics can you maximize your comfort and increase your chances of success.

RACE DAY CHECKLIST

Before leaving home for your next marathon, use a checklist such as this one to make certain you have not forgotten any essential items. This list was developed by Ron Gunn, dean of sports medicine at Southwestern Michigan College, when we led groups of runners on tours to races such as the Honolulu Marathon.

CARRY-ON LUGGAGE
Racing shoes
Travel itinerary
Airline tickets
Toiletries
Passport and other documents
Credit cards
Toothbrush and toothpaste
Camera and film
Hotel and rental car confirmation
Wallet and money
Event information

OTHER GEAR
Dress clothes
Race socks
Dress shoes
Throwaway cold-weather gear
Socks
Warmup suit
Underwear
Swimsuit
Coat

(continued)

Cap

Gloves

Safety pins

Rain gear

Body lubricant

Sunglasses

Tape and adhesive bandages

Sunscreen

Medicine

Alarm clock

Favorite race drink

Race uniform

21

Drinking on the Run

What and When to Drink

Paths along the Chicago lakefront stretch 18 miles from the South Shore Cultural Center on the South Side to Bryn Mawr Avenue on the North Side, encompassing Jackson, Grant, and Lincoln Parks. When you run on the lakefront, you encounter museums, one of the largest convention centers in the world, the football stadium where the Chicago Bears play, high-rise apartments, a lift bridge, several yacht clubs and golf courses, and numerous sandy beaches jammed each summer with swimmers.

Most important, there are water fountains—a total of thirty-two of them, according to one map used by runners to plan their workouts. And each summer as the local training classes do their long runs to prepare for the Chicago Marathon, runners stop frequently to drink. It is our means of survival. But survival is merely one reason that runners need to drink when they run far. The other reasons are to replace lost energy, enhance performance, and prevent cramps, perhaps related to dehydration, that sometimes strike in the last miles of a marathon.

Before running became a mass participation affair, runners ignored fluids while running marathons because of a combination of arrogance, ignorance, and a lack of aid stations. Scientists and running writers like me had not yet spread the news that proper fluid replacement can make you run faster. Emil Zatopek, the great Czech runner, won the 1952 Olympic marathon without taking a sip! But today's runners know how to drink. They drink often—water as well as replacement fluids, which are marketed these days as aggressively as soft drinks.

At a nutrition seminar at Ohio State University in Columbus before the 1992 Olympic trials, Edward F. Coyle, PhD, of the department of kinesiology at the University of Texas at Austin, suggested that for efficient thermal regulation on a hot day, a runner who loses 1 kilogram (2.2 pounds) an hour would need to drink at least 1,000 milliliters of fluid an hour. That is a full liter—nearly 1 quart!—and more than most runners voluntarily consume. That is why you want to learn your sweat rate—so you can replace fluids according to your personal needs. By weighing yourself without clothing before and after a 1-hour run at race pace (keeping in mind varying air temperatures), you can determine how much sweat you lose. One pound of weight lost equates to 16 ounces of sweat lost; 2 pounds equates to 1 quart.

Clydesdales sweat more than lightweight runners, and some runners sweat heavily while others barely glow. If you are a 4- or 5-hour marathoner who sweats heavily and loses 2 pounds (32 ounces, or 1 quart) an hour, you might need to drink 4 or 5 quart bottles of fluid. You are unlikely to do that without *programmed drinking*— that is, drinking 8 ounces every 15 minutes to replace sweat losses.

THE THINKING ON DRINKING

In the first two editions of this book, I encouraged runners to "drink, drink, drink." I modified that statement for later editions, suggesting only that runners learn to "drink on the run." The thinking on drinking has changed. Runners who walk around at expos the day before their marathons, sipping from plastic bottles, may now be drinking too much. Many major marathons with five-figure fields offer aid stations nearly every mile as one means of coping with the crowding. You can drown out there!

Excessive hydration may get you in trouble, today's experts believe. "Drinking too little is common," concedes Amby Burfoot of *Runner's World*, "but drinking too much is more dangerous." Drinking too little is a performance issue: It slows you down. Drinking too much can sometimes kill you because of a condition known as hyponatremia, caused by excessive fluid consumption.

Many people believe they need to drink eight 8-ounce glasses of water a day because some fashion magazine told them so. But no scientific research exists to support the 8 × 8 thesis, wrote Burfoot in the July 2003 issue of *Runner's World*.

"Dehydration diminishes performance," Burfoot stated, "because it thickens the blood, decreases the heart's efficiency, increases heart rate, and raises body temperature. But a modest dehydration is a normal and temporary condition for many marathoners and doesn't lead to any serious medical conditions. Excessive fluid consumption, on the other hand, can prove deadly."

The problem is not so much the elites, who run so fast that organizers need to provide them with special tables for their own water bottles. They are off the course in just over 2 hours. It is more the increasing number of slower runners, who may be running under the sun for 5 or 6 hours. They can drink all they want while walking past the numerous aid stations. That many of these runners are women compounds the problem, says Burfoot, because women need only 70 percent as much fluid as men due to lesser body mass.

(continued)

Hyponatremia means low blood sodium. Excessive fluid consumption lowers the concentration of sodium in the blood. In extreme cases, hyponatremia can cause death through brain seizures, which has happened at several marathons. As a result, organizations such as the International Marathon Medical Directors Association have changed their recommended race fluid consumption guidelines: Drink to thirst.

Stay hydrated, goes the current advice, but do not overdrink. Maybe you need to skip a few of those aid stations. I can't give you a precise number, because we are all different. (Too many variables.) Nevertheless, sports drinks that contain at least some sodium may offer you an extra dose of protection.

HOW TO DRINK

The leaders of the Chicago Marathon training classes encourage participants to drink freely during their runs. Not only does drinking fluids make their weekend long runs more comfortable, but it teaches them how to drink and how often to drink. No tennis player would start a match without practicing lobs; no golfer would think a game complete without learning how to pitch from a sand trap. And no runner should enter a marathon without figuring out how, how much, and when to drink.

Drinking while running definitely is not easy. Unless you grasp the cup carefully, you can spill half the contents on the ground. If you gulp too quickly, you can spend the next mile coughing and gasping. If you dawdle at aid stations, you can waste precious seconds. If you gulp down a replacement drink you are not used to, it may make you nauseated. Lately, scientists have suggested that drinking too much during a marathon sometimes can be as dangerous on a hot day as drinking too little, because it can result in hyponatremia. Finding the balance between too much and too little is not easy, but who ever said running a marathon was easy?

Drinking on the run is necessary for survival. When the weather is warm or humid, runners sweat. You sweat even during cool weather, particularly if you are overdressed. If you sweat too much, you dehydrate. If you become dehydrated, your body temperature rises and performance drops. Too high a body temperature can result in heat prostration or—in extreme circumstances—death.

Most people sweat efficiently and adapt quite well to changes in temperature. It is why humans occupy the Earth, while dinosaurs are seen only in scary movies. It is only when you undertake extreme activities such as marathons that you need to worry about taking in enough liquid to balance losses from sweat. The average sedentary person loses 2 quarts of water a day under normal temperature conditions, but a marathoner can sweat away that much in half an hour, according to Lawrence E. Armstrong, PhD, of the University of Connecticut, who included among his specialties the study of dehydration.

Drinking while running definitely is not easy.

Some people sweat very little; some sweat a lot. Alberto Salazar, for example, lost 12 pounds and finished a subpar fifteenth in the 1984 Olympic marathon, which he ran in the warm conditions of Los Angeles.

Nevertheless, sweating is a natural result of exercise. As we run, every muscle operates like a miniature furnace producing an excess of heat. The resulting rise in body temperature triggers the production and excretion of sweat through the body's sweat glands. As sweat evaporates from the skin, you cool off. This process is called *thermoregulation*, and when it works right, it serves as an effective heating and cooling system.

Unfortunately for those of us running marathons, what scientists refer to as effective thermoregulation occurs at the expense of body fluids. The hotter it is, the more you sweat. "If sweat loss is not replaced during exercise," warns Robert Murray, PhD, of Sports Science Insights, "the resulting dehydration compromises cardiovascular and thermoregulatory function, increases the risk of heat illness, and impairs exercise performance."

Dehydration reduces blood volume. This prompts the body to decrease both blood flow and sweating in an attempt to conserve body fluids. Under these circumstances, the body's ability to cool itself declines, and body temperature can rise to dangerous levels unless you stop running—and it may not decrease even then if you fail to get out of the sun.

You cannot adapt to dehydration, but living and training in hot environments can help you avoid or at least delay dehydration. Want to become a better hot-weather runner? Move to Africa. As you adapt to warmer climates, your blood volume expands and your sweat glands conserve sodium. "This helps assure that cardiovascular and thermoregulatory function can be maintained during exercise in the heat," says Dr. Murray.

> **Want to become a better hot-weather runner? Move to Africa.**

In other words, we can train ourselves to use fluids more efficiently. Humans are homeotherms who need to maintain a constant temperature; we are warm-blooded rather than cold-blooded. An internal temperature of 98.6°F is considered normal. When the nurse at the doctor's office measures your temperature, that is the number he or she wants to see. Your body temperature drops below normal (called *hypothermia*) if you stay out in the cold too long or wear insufficient clothing. Your temperature rises above normal (*hyperthermia*) when you start to exercise. It also rises if you get the flu or a similar infection, one reason it is not a good idea to exercise to excess—or even at all—when you are ill. Hypothermia normally is not a major problem for marathoners, except occasionally on cold days when runners may feel less urge to drink. If forced to slow down because of fatigue or dehydration, they may experience a drop in body temperature. This happens sometimes to runners in the Boston Marathon who reach the top of Heartbreak Hill, fatigued, and suddenly encounter cool winds off the ocean. (Drinking helps keep you warm as well as cool, as I have discovered while competing in cross-country ski races.)

PREVENTING MUSCLE CRAMPS

Marathoners often experience muscle cramps—in the calves, the stomach, and various other body parts—about 18 or 20 miles into a marathon. Conventional wisdom suggests that dehydration and the loss of various electrolytes—specifically, sodium—causes cramps. Sometimes this is true, but not always.

Nutritionist Nancy Clark writes: "Muscle cramps are often associated with dehydration. If you have ever experienced the excruciating pain of a severe muscle cramp, you may fearfully wonder whether it will strike again. Unfortunately, no one totally understands what causes muscle cramps, but if you've had one, you are at risk for having more." Clark suggests that fatigue may be more a factor than scientists in the past believed.

E. Randy Eichner, MD, of the University of Oklahoma Medical Center and a member of the *Runner's World* Science Advisory Board, agrees while saying the three root causes of heat cramping are salt loss, dehydration, and muscle fatigue. "Sodium is a key," says Dr. Eichner, "not only to maintain blood volume but also to help nerves fire and muscles work. Sodium depletion short-circuits the coordination of nerves and muscles as muscles contract and relax." The result, he says, can be muscle cramping. Cramps are painful and can impede performances, but they can also be one of the signs of hypothermia. While no cure-all exists for cramps, these strategies may help prevent them in your next race.

1. Train properly for your marathon, especially with long runs that build strength and muscle endurance.

(continued)

2. Balance your diet with a good mix of fruits and vegetables and other foods that contain the vitamins and minerals you need—specifically, sodium, potassium, magnesium, and calcium.

3. Before a long run, eat something salty, such as soup, salted crackers, or salted oatmeal; this helps your body retain water.

4. Learn to drink during the marathon—preferably a sports drink containing sodium—but do not drink excessively, including before the race. The sodium in a sports drink is added primarily to enhance fluid retention; it is not enough to replace sweat loss of sodium.

5. Check your biomechanics. If poor form or a poor foot plant places extra stress on certain muscles, those muscles may cramp more easily.

6. Include stretching in your training routine. Your muscles need to be loose as well as strong.

7. Salt tablets (a quick source of sodium) may work for heavy sweaters. Experiment with extra salt during long training runs before trying it in a marathon. Drink at least 8 ounces of water with each tablet.

When and if you do cramp, what can you do to relieve the pain? Craig A. Horswill, PhD, a senior research fellow at the Gatorade Sports Science Institute, recommends both stretching and massaging the complaining muscles. "Rubbing the cramped muscle may help alleviate pain as well as stimulate bloodflow and fluid movement into the area," says Dr. Horswill.

Hyperthermia is more of a problem. Even though we begin sweating almost immediately as a response to exercise, it may be 10 minutes or more before skin becomes noticeably moist. On hot but dry days, you may not realize you are sweating because the moisture evaporates quickly.

Sweat is normally very dilute, containing only about 10 percent electrolytes—mostly sodium chloride and some potassium. Cooling occurs when sweat evaporates from the body surface. Evaporation is important. Blood flows to the surface and transfers its heat by conduction.

During exercise, the body usually produces more heat than you can get rid of by sweating. A marathoner's body temperature gradually rises 3°F or 4°F to 102°F, an efficient level for energy use. At this point, your air-conditioning system is in sync with the environment, and you perform well. If the weather is too hot or too humid or you become dehydrated—resulting in a drop in sweat production—the body's temperature can soar to dangerous levels. Your muscles will not perform efficiently at temperatures that are too high (104°F and up), so that will slow you down. This is an important defense mechanism, because if you fail to sweat and your core temperature rises much past 106°F, you may experience heatstroke, a serious problem for which the early symptoms are headaches and dizziness, followed in extreme cases by convulsions, unconsciousness, and death.

When heatstroke occurs, the only sane approach—excuse the language—is to get the hell off the course! That assumes that the dehydrated runner recognizes his or her body signals to stop running.

The body's ability to safely regulate its internal temperature while exercising is influenced by four factors: the environment, exercise intensity, clothing, and the athlete's level of fitness and acclimatization. You can train yourself to resist both cold and hot weather, but extremes of either can cause problems.

Conditioning will improve your ability to sweat. The late Carl Gisolfi, PhD, an exercise physiologist at the University of Iowa, believed that we can increase our heat tolerance 50 percent by conditioning. According to Dr. Gisolfi, you train your sweat glands to function more efficiently by using them.

Acclimatization also improves the body's ability to tolerate heat. That is why marathoners experience more problems when the weather turns hot at Boston in April than at New York in the fall. By New York, they have had an entire summer to become acclimatized.

Former world record holder Buddy Edelen, a graduate of the University of Minnesota, sometimes wore three sweat suits to simulate hot conditions while training for the 1964 Olympic marathon trials. Sure enough, temperatures rose into the 90s during the May trials in Yonkers, New York, and Edelen soundly beat his rivals. Later, Olympic marathoners Ron Daws of Minnesota and Benji Durden of Colorado adopted Edelen's training strategy of keeping very hot temperatures in mind with success, as did Deena Drossin Kastor, bronze medalist at the 2004 Olympic Games in Athens. On a frighteningly hot day in August, while many of her rivals were outdoors warming up on a track, Deena stayed indoors, keeping her body temperature low by wearing an ice vest developed by one of her sponsors. That leads to my next point.

STAY COOL

Other than training in multiple sweat suits or purchasing ice vests, what strategies can runners use to prevent heat problems? Let us talk first about training. Here are some training tips for proper hydration.

DRINK BEFORE RUNNING

Drink adequately and drink often. Dr. Murray recommends drinking 16 ounces of water an hour before training. "Excess body water will be passed as urine before practice begins," he says. The one caution I would offer is that if you drink too much—particularly before an important race—you may need to waste time ducking into a portable toilet. Knowing how much to drink and when is something to determine during long workouts, and maybe in races leading to your marathon. Sports nutritionist Nancy Clark suggests you time your drinking to learn how long it takes for water to go in one end and out the other. I might drink an hour before a workout but would not chance that short a time frame before a marathon.

DRINK WHILE YOU RUN

For years, an old-fashioned notion among football coaches was that drinking was for sissies. They prohibited their athletes from going near water fountains during summer practices. Today's more knowledgeable coaches realize their athletes practice and play better if allowed time to drink. That was the motivation behind the development of Gatorade, a replacement drink formulated for University of Florida football players (the Gators). Runners need to drink frequently while training, especially during warm weather. You will run faster and recover faster. Most runners quickly become adept at locating available water in their neighborhoods. I sometimes carry money in my shorts if I know I'll be passing a soft drink machine.

WALK TO DRINK

In preparing for the marathon at the 1981 World Masters Championships in Christchurch, New Zealand, I experimented with walking through aid stations at several shorter races and discovered I lost only 7 seconds off my time if I walked to drink at each aid station. That is inconsequential. In the race, I walked through every aid station (positioned at 5K intervals) and figured I lost less than a minute en route to victory in the M45 age group with a time of 2:29:27. Many of the runners I beat that day had posted faster times coming into the race but finished behind me on a warm day. (I had outthunk them and outdrunk them!)

If a front-runner loses only 7 seconds each time he walks through an aid station running at a 5:30 pace, you will lose even less running time at a slower pace. When I lead 4:30 pacing groups at marathons, we average 10:18 per mile. Most fit runners can walk 15:00 per mile or faster, so the drop-off between running pace and walking pace is small, but the gain is great. Stopping to drink, however, can be an antisocial act if it results in your blocking following runners from the table.

DRINK AFTER RUNNING

Most runners do not need to be told this. Their natural instinct sends them immediately to the water fountain or refrigerator. But even after your initial thirst is quenched, you still may be dehydrated. One way of evaluating your intake is to check the color of your urine. If it is dark yellow (or you fail to produce urine), you probably need to keep drinking. Clear urine is a sign of good hydration. Another clue is body weight. If your weight is abnormally low after a long run on a hot day, do not congratulate yourself that you are losing weight; you are most likely badly dehydrated. Particularly after long runs, it is a good idea to drink more than just water. Low-fat chocolate milk is an excellent recovery beverage. Better than a sports drink, it provides more carbs to help replenish glycogen burned during your run, more protein to heal damaged muscles, and more sodium and other minerals to replace electrolytes. You will recover much more rapidly and help prevent injuries if you drink chocolate milk.

RUN WHEN IT IS COOL

Because of my flexible schedule as a writer, I always have been able to choose my running times. During the winter, I usually trained at midday because it was warmer. During the summer, I switched to running at dawn, before it got too hot. Running in the evening is slightly less satisfactory because it can still be hot and humid. And running in the dark has its own perils.

You may need to do some hot-weather running to acclimatize yourself for races, but you do not want extreme temperatures to affect the quality of your training. I have run at 4:00 in the afternoon near my brother-in-law's house in Mesa, Arizona, when the temperature was 104°F. I did not run far and I did not run fast, but I ran—partly to prove I could do it. I was glad I did not have to run in those conditions every day.

SHIFT YOUR TRAINING

The message in one of my earlier books, *Run Fast*, was this: "If you want to run fast, you have to run fast." Every coach will tell you that one secret to success—even in the marathon—is speedwork. The best time for speedwork is the summer, when the warm weather helps warm your muscles so you are less likely to experience injuries. You can train on the track, never more than a short sprint from a water fountain or a bottle stashed on the infield grass. Short, intense workouts can get you just as hot as long, slow ones, but you will be closer to home if you do overheat.

BEWARE OF THE SUN

Wear a hat. Every runner should own a sloppy, floppy hat that can be used to douse yourself with water when you stop at water fountains. There are some excellent runners' hats now that are made of lightweight, breathable materials. You may want to use sunscreen (for best results, use a sun protection factor, or SPF, of 15 or higher) to protect vulnerable areas, such as your face, your shoulders, and the fronts of your legs. Apply the sunscreen half an hour before you run to give it time to dry and be absorbed, then apply more. Layering works with sunscreen as much as layering clothing when it is cold. Wash your hands thoroughly to avoid rubbing the lotion into your eyes if you wipe your face; it can sting badly. For the same reason, you may want to apply the lotion only below your eyes, trusting your cap to protect your forehead.

I cannot overstate the importance of running covered when the sun is strong. Always—and I mean always—run with a hat when the sun is high overhead, specifically between 10:00 a.m. and 2:00 p.m.

DO NOT OVERESTIMATE YOUR ABILITY

Realize that you cannot run as fast when it is warm. Learn your limits. Do not expect to achieve a planned time, and do not be afraid to bail out early when you are starting to overheat.

I learned that lesson the hard way. During the prime of my running career, I set out foolishly one morning determined to run at a 5:30 pace on a long run of 23 miles without realizing that the temperature was climbing through the 80s. I finished the workout, but was barely jogging. Two days later, I came down with a knee injury, which I attributed to my still-dehydrated state. You cannot ignore Mother Nature while running in the heat. Warm-weather training must of necessity be a compromise. But if you learn to live with the heat, you can survive and condition yourself for any type of weather.

MARATHON MEALS

Unlike cyclists and skiers, most fast marathoners avoid solid foods when they run, for a simple reason: It is difficult to eat while moving at a fast pace. (I'll let you define what is "fast pace.")

But Coach Bill Wenmark recommends midmarathon snacks for people who take much longer than 3 hours to finish. "If you're on the road for 4 or 5 hours, you're running the equivalent of an ultramarathon," says Wenmark. "You need more energy than you can get from the drinks race directors provide. Someone running an 8:00 pace or slower can take time to eat. Digestion is less of a problem for them than for elite runners." Wenmark recommends saltines and energy bars for his back-of-the-packers, and he positions support crews along the course to provide this extra boost.

What do the scientists say? At Ohio State University, W. Michael Sherman, PhD, an exercise scientist, tested ten cyclists who rode at 70 percent of their maximum capacity for 90 minutes, then did the equivalent of a 20-mile time trial. (Their total time approached 2½ hours.) In one trial they ate a specific amount of carbohydrates, and in the other they got the carbs in liquid form. "We found no performance difference in their response," reports Dr. Sherman. He adds that in warm weather, liquids certainly would be preferable to solids because the fluids would help combat dehydration.

Dr. Sherman notes that his study did not explore the outer realm of endurance beyond 4 and 5 hours, where ultramarathoners (and slow marathoners) tread. Conventional wisdom among this breed suggests that food may be as important as drink—if only for the psychological reason that you want something solid in your stomach. Slower marathoners seem to have a stronger desire to eat solid food than experienced marathoners, who have adapted to a liquid-only diet while racing. Liquids high in sugar (such as gels) can sometimes cause stomach distress—nausea and diarrhea—if you are not used to them or consume too many of them during an event.

Until recently, few American marathons provided anything other than liquids. If you wanted food and were unwilling to carry what you wanted in a fanny pack, you needed to enlist a support crew. Lately, manufacturers have provided gels and sports candies that can be carried easily in a pocket or pinned to a singlet, as well as banana chunks, hard candy, mini chocolate bars, and other carb-rich options. Standard foods do the job just as well as commercial sports foods.

The most innovative food option in my many marathons, I thought, was in the Comrades Marathon, a 50-plus-mile race between Durban and Pietermaritzburg in South Africa: baked potatoes! A close second was the Kosice Peace Marathon in Czechoslovakia: soup with chunks of something floating in it. I passed on the soup because of my self-imposed rule that you never do anything new in a marathon.

Most important: If you plan to eat on the run, experiment often in practice before you race.

Still, it is sometimes difficult to gauge the weather. My oldest son, Kevin, qualified for the 1984 Olympic marathon trials with a time of

2:18:50. He was not a threat to make the top three, but the level of his training suggested that he might be able to shave several minutes off that PR in the trials race, which began in Buffalo, New York, and finished at Niagara Falls, Ontario. As his coach, I designed an even pace to achieve that goal. Carefully watching his splits, Kevin cruised past 10 miles right on pace, but he had to drop out a half dozen miles later because that pace was too fast for the hot and humid conditions, which we had failed to recognize at the start. Meanwhile, the runners at the front of the pack ran against one another, not against their watches, and had far fewer problems—although their times were several minutes slower than might have been expected.

Conditioning will improve your ability to sweat.

As a leader of pacing teams at various marathons, I would warn runners of the danger of connecting with a team that is too fast, particularly on a hot or humid day. At the prerace clinics, I usually advise those who planned to join the 4:00 team to move back to the 4:10 or 4:20 team. Those planning 4:10 finishes move back to 4:20 or 4:30, and so forth. But runners often come to marathons programmed to run specific times. It is sometimes difficult to accept that despite all your hard training, you are not going to achieve your time goal because of the environment.

REFUEL ON THE RUN

Drinking during a marathon is almost a separate subject because in addition to your need to stay cool, you need to adopt a strategy that permits you to refuel on the run. You need energy as well as fluid replacement. Sports drinks offer both. Learn what beverages will be available by checking the race's website, then practice with that drink during long distance runs.

Timing your prerace hydration can be tricky. I recommend that runners drink up until about 2 hours before the race. This allows plenty of time to process and eliminate the excess, often in the comfort of your hotel bathroom. Otherwise, you may need to urinate at midrace, an obvious inconvenience. After these 2 hours of abstinence, drink again just before the pack around you starts to move. (In large races, this can be several minutes after the gun sounds.) Every runner needs to experiment and come up with a workable drinking routine before practice and before races.

Once across the starting line, you should begin drinking early in the race. If you wait until you get thirsty, you may already have passed several aid stations that could have helped you avoid dehydration. Because of the crowds in the early miles, it may be difficult to get near the aid station for your first drink. But that drink may be the most important one you take in the race; it is worth losing a few seconds to grab at least a cup of water. One tip to remember is that it may be less crowded at the end tables of the aid station than at the first tables. Another is to remember that right-handed runners may often gravitate to tables to the right of the course. Unfortunately, I have offered this advice so often in earlier editions that runners who read the first four editions of this book may crowd you away from the left-side tables.

But the important goal is staying cool. "Any dehydration causes problems," says Dr. Coyle. "None can be tolerated." This is true not only in terms of safety but also in terms of performance. For every liter of fluid you lose, your heartbeat will increase 8 beats per minute and your core temperature will increase accordingly. As a result, you will be unable to maintain your race pace. If your goal is safety and performance, there is no question that the closer you match your intake of fluids to your rate of dehydration, the better.

THE 6 PERCENT SOLUTION

Early research in fluid replacement suggested that drinks high in sugar content emptied from the stomach more slowly than water. Then scientists fine-tuned their experiments and determined that fluids with a 6 percent sugar solution emptied from the stomach almost as fast as water, which is preferable because you want those fluids to get to the areas of the body where they're most needed. Most replacement drinks now offered at major marathons are formulated at that level. So do not bypass the replacement drink at aid stations (unless the sugar in the drink makes you nauseated).

My approach is usually to grab the replacement drink first, then wash it down with water, although some marathons offer water first, replacement drink second. Temperature usually dictates how much of each I drink. In warmer weather, I shade the ratio more toward water. I've found that too much replacement drink causes stomach problems for me, but everyone is different in this respect.

Edward F. Coyle, PhD, of the department of kinesiology at the University of Texas at Austin, estimates that ingesting 30 to 60 grams of carbohydrates with each hour of exercise will generally help you maintain blood glucose oxidation late in exercise and delay fatigue.

You can reach this level by drinking between 625 and 1,250 milliliters (about ⅔ quart to 1¼ quarts) per hour of a beverage that contains between 4 percent and 8 percent carbohydrates. For races beyond the marathon distance, when energy replacement becomes as important as thermoregulation, consuming food (dried fruit, chocolate, a peanut butter and jelly sandwich, banana bread—whatever you can tolerate) can be helpful. Research by Asker Jeukendrup of the University of Birmingham in England suggests that ingesting up to 90 grams of carbs (360 calories) per hour optimizes endurance.

In the closing stages of the race, water splashed on the body may help you more than water taken into the body. This is because it normally takes 10 to 30 minutes for water to migrate through your system to be released as sweat and provide an air-conditioning effect. One way to shortcut that system is to pour water directly on your body, permitting it to evaporate. In the last few miles of the race, you are drinking for recovery after the race as much as for performance during it. My motto for the last half hour of running is "Water on" as much as "Water in." Some scientists suggest that splashing water on your body will not cool you significantly. Maybe so, but it sure feels good—and the psychological boost is worth something.

If you are wearing a hat, pour water onto it and let the water drip onto your face. Rather than splashing yourself in front, pour water down your back, so it is less likely to flow down into your shoes and cause blisters. If you pass someone standing beside the road with a water spray, consider stopping to stand under the spray for at least a few seconds rather than running through or around it.

The more attention you give to staying cool, the better you will run. Once you get across the finish line, you will want to begin drinking immediately to speed your recovery, but that is a subject for another chapter.

22

Mind Games

Running Is a Mental as Well as Physical Sport

Even in early October, the Twin Cities Marathon, held between Minneapolis and St. Paul, can be chilly. One year, with the temperature just below freezing at the 7:00 a.m. start, I came prepared, wearing tights, a long-sleeved top, a hat, and gloves. Having attended college in Minnesota, I knew what to expect. Unfortunately, on the way to the starting line, I lost one of the gloves. To keep both hands warm as I ran, I switched the lone glove from hand to hand every third mile. It became a game for me, something to think about, something to help chart my progress. I could look forward to the switch every 3 miles.

If you think in those terms, a marathon is merely eight glove changes long.

Psychologists have long insisted that the mind is as important as the body when it comes to success in sports, particularly in an event like the marathon, where the mind must push the body to extremes. During the glory days of Eastern Bloc athletes, sports psychologists were as important as other coaches or trainers in preparing East German and Soviet athletes for competition. The U.S. Olympic Committee employs psychologists as consultants, as do many professional football and baseball teams. But anyone can use mind games to help get themselves through long-distance events.

I use mind games for survival in the marathon, physically as well as mentally. I divide marathons into fourths and thirds. At 3 miles I think: *Just done a 5K. Piece of cake.* At 6 miles it's: *A fourth of the race done.* And at 8 miles: *A third.* At 10 miles I console myself: *Double digits.* At 13 miles: *Past the half. Fewer miles ahead than behind.* At 16 miles: *Only single digits remain.* At 20 miles: *I've passed the wall* or *Only 10K left now.* By that time, you're close enough to count down like the liftoff of a rocket: *Six-five-four-three-two-one. I'm done.*

Actually, I like international marathons better than those in the United States because kilometer markings allow you to count down more often: "Ten-nine-eight-seven-six-five-four-three-two-one."

The mind is as important as the body when it comes to success in sports.

Carolyn Warren of Tinley Park, Illinois, takes a slightly different approach, dividing the marathon into approximately 2-mile increments; it is simply thirteen aid station stops. As marathoners, we play various mind games to get ourselves to finish 26 miles 385 yards as fast as possible.

"Every marathon experience is different," says Cindy Southgate of Kanata, Ontario. "You need to figure out which mind games will work for that particular day."

While researching *Boston: A Century of Running* before the classic 100th anniversary race in 1996, I interviewed Dick Beardsley, who finished second to Alberto Salazar at the 1982 race. Coming off Heartbreak Hill in the lead but with Salazar stalking him, Beardsley was toast. At 21 miles, he decided to adopt a strategy that ignored the fact that 5 grueling miles remained. He decided he would run those miles one at a time, not caring whether there was another mile, not worrying whether there would be a tomorrow. "You can hold this pace for 1 more mile," Beardsley told himself. "One more mile! Only 1 mile to go!"

At 22 miles, Beardsley punched the reset button on his mental speed-ometer. "One mile to go!"

And at 23 miles: "You're beating the world record holder. One more mile!" Salazar eventually did outsprint Beardsley on the final straight-away, beating him 2:08:52 to 2:08:54. But it was Beardsley's mental strength that made their duel one of the closest races in Boston Mara-thon history.

I have adopted that strategy in several races, including one year at the Disney World Marathon, in which I led the 4:30 pacing team for *Runner's World*. I arrived in Orlando undertrained, having failed to do any work-outs beyond 13 miles in the months before the race. Though in respect-able shape for a 5K or a 10K, I doubted my ability to keep the pace for a full 26. I told my co-leader that I planned to go only 20, then she could take the group the rest of the way.

But at 20 I felt okay, so I tucked in behind the group, focused on the ears of the Mickey Mouse cap my co-leader was wearing, and told my-self, "One mile to go. You can hold this pace for 1 more mile!" And like Beardsley, I reset my mental speedometer for each of the next half dozen miles. Although the group did pull ahead by 40 seconds in those closing miles, I finished in 4:30:27. That gave me more satisfaction than many races in which my times were several hours faster.

POSITIVE THINKING

Marathon mind games are more than strategies for coping with pain and boredom. According to Charles A. Garfield, author of *Peak Performance*, 60 percent to 90 percent of success in sports can be attributed to mental fac-tors and psychological mastery. Sports psychologist Thomas Tutko, PhD, quotes retired baseball player Maury Wills as saying that success is all mental. "There is nothing mystical about the emotional side of sports," claims Dr. Tutko.

Unfortunately, your mind can also work against you. One individual commented to me about a top-ranked female runner he formerly coached: "It's her thinking that keeps her from winning."

Confidence remains an important factor—when we are confident, we can rationalize away any potential problems. Without confidence, even slight threats become magnified.

Confident athletes can relax more easily than ones who feel threatened, but there are tricks to relaxing and eliminating fear. Olympic marathoner Tony Sandoval used a five-to-zero countdown when he went to bed each night. "It relaxed me and helped me fall asleep quickly," explains Sandoval.

As a steeplechaser, I had my own pre-sleep technique. I would visualize myself hurdling over barriers. It was better, I thought, than the more traditional counting of sheep, but it served another purpose beyond self-hypnosis. I was perfecting my hurdling technique through a method known as imaging. Marathoners can practice a similar technique, mentally reviewing the course before a race and thinking about how they will run it.

Sixty percent to 90 percent of success in sports can be attributed to mental factors.

One way to succeed in sports is to eliminate outside distractions. Concentration continues to be a key to success for fast runners and should be for midpack runners, too. "The ability to concentrate," says William P. Morgan, EdD, a sports psychologist at the University of Wisconsin at Madison, "is the single element that separates the merely good athletes from the great ones. Concentration is the hallmark of the elite runner." Elite runners succeed, he says, because they are totally in tune with their bodies, monitoring all symptoms from the nerve endings.

In contrast, Dr. Morgan found that midpack marathoners more often thought of another activity (called dissociating) as a means of coping with pain. Dr. Morgan believes that in addition to possibly slowing them down, this tactic is dangerous: "Runners could be ignoring important body signals and mindlessly run themselves into heatstroke or a stress fracture." Although dissociation blocks negative messages, it can block positive messages, too. For that reason, listening to music while running may unnecessarily distract you from the task at hand. Particularly at large races, I recommend leaving your music player at home because you will miss a lot of the fun going on around you.

MIDPACK MIND GAMES

Although scientists suggest that tightly focusing on the task at hand (associating) allows elite athletes to extract the last ounce of energy from their bodies and win the race, midpack athletes often find themselves faced with a different challenge. They seek any strategy that will allow them to finish the race in a respectable time.

North Carolinian Don Pocock, whose PR is 3:38, has a series of strategies, including a mantra, that he uses when he runs marathons. The mantra is "Go the distance," which he chants repeatedly. "My track coach gave it to us back in high school to motivate us," Pocock recalls. "I now use the chant to keep my mind occupied with something else when every muscle in my body is screaming 'Stop!'"

Pocock also spells words as another diversion. "Sometimes I get a sentence or a phrase in my mind and work it over and over to pass time," he says. "Sometimes I even go over Russian vocabulary just to have something different to think about."

Finally, near the end of the marathon, Pocock pictures friends or family cheering him on, even if they are not there. "It works pretty well," he says, "and folks usually like to hear that you were thinking about them during the race."

Kazuo Takai of the University of Tsukuba split sixty runners into groups at a 20K race in Tokyo. Half the runners used what Takai described as "attention" techniques to stay on pace; half used "avoidance" techniques and followed the pace of the others. Takai found that the attentive runners outperformed the avoidance runners in achieving their predicted goals. Attention means that you tune in to your body's signals midrace and let how you feel dictate your pace. Avoidance means that you tune out your body's signals and go with the flow.

Does this mean that joining a pacing team is a form of avoidance? It depends on your goals and how you hope to achieve them by joining a team. Yes, if you let the team leader do all the work for you. No, if you focus tightly on staying with the leader, monitoring closely how successful he or she is at keeping you on pace. That could be considered a form of attention. Avoidance is not always a losing strategy, however, and some pacing team members may choose avoidance at some points of the race and attention at other times.

Takai's spin on the subject was to identify five attention strategies that contributed to good race times.

1. **Body check.** How does your whole body feel? Are you loose and relaxed? Any tight spots (such as a sore shoulder) may be a signal to slow down.

2. **Tempo test.** How is the rhythm of your running? Do you feel smo-o-o-th? You should flow along the ground as though this were an easy practice run.

3. **Leg rest.** Can your legs continue to carry you at this pace? Any cramps? Discomfort? Maybe by speeding up, you will actually feel more comfortable.

4. **Image replay.** Remember your most successful races or practice runs. Do you feel as well now as you did then? Recapture the glory by picturing past triumphs.

5. **Motion study.** Are you running well? Move out of your own body and see yourself as though through a video camera. Now improve that picture.

Takai asked each of his subjects to indicate on a 7-point rating scale (1 = never; 7 = very often) how often they used these strategies to recall pace in a race. He then compared how close the runners came to their predicted time in a 5K. This enabled him to rate them as "accurate" or "inaccurate" recallers. Results showed that the accurate recallers were better pacers, capable of running steady through the race. "Overall," says Takai, "the accurate recallers ran with a steady pace throughout the race, while the inaccurate recallers were likely to decrease the pace after the first 5K."

Maintaining a steady pace or even having the energy to pick up the pace late in the race can be an effective strategy, since you will pass a lot of runners in the last half-dozen miles who went out too fast. Deena Drossin Kastor applied that approach in winning a bronze medal at the 2004 Olympic Games. "The smartest way to race is to pick off runners," she commented after her third-place finish. "I started to get an adrenaline rush every time I saw another girl in front of me."

> One way to succeed in sports is to eliminate outside distractions.

When I ran marathons near the front of the pack, I always considered concentration to be as important an ability as a high VO$_2$ max. I focused on every stride and was acutely aware of any signals my body was sending. I always liked the idea of running on scenic courses—except I almost never saw the scenery! Usually the better I ran, the less I recalled of the surroundings. I had run the Boston Marathon ten times and knew that the course passed somewhere near Fenway Park, where the Boston Red Sox play, but I was unaware how near until one year in the 1970s when I first covered the race for *Runner's World* as a journalist. After the lead runners had finished,

I decided to wander back over the course to watch the remaining runners. Less than a mile from the finish line, I came upon Fenway Park. I was startled. Intellectually, I had realized that Fenway was right on the course, but I had never seen it before. For me to have missed it while racing, my field of vision must have been very narrow.

THE VALUE OF CONCENTRATION

Other runners agree on the value of concentration. Olympic marathoner Don Kardong states, "It's absolutely essential that you concentrate on your competition, monitor your body feedback, and not lose touch with what's happening around you. If you lose concentration in a good, competitive 10,000-meter race, you immediately drop off the pace. There's never time to think those favorite thoughts you have on easy training runs."

Greg Meyer, who struggled to regain his form after winning Boston in 1983, ran several meets in Europe one summer. "I'd lose concentration for a lap or two," Meyer told me, "and that would get me out of the race. I'd drift off, get gapped, and never make it up."

Meyer felt that a series of injuries contributed to his inability to concentrate. "You start focusing on the injuries instead of racing," he said. But it was possible that in winning Boston, he had satisfied many of the inner demons that had driven him to success. He may have lost some of his will to win and, with it, the ability to concentrate.

Kardong notes that some distance runners have difficulty switching from roads to track or cross-country. He suspects that the biggest factor is not training but concentration: "When in an unfamiliar setting, you're distracted by it initially. Later, you adapt."

During a marathon, Bill Rodgers would think of specific things to help him concentrate: splits, competition, the course, the wind. If he had a chance to win, he thought: *What's my best way to race certain individuals?*

Meyer learned he could concentrate better in training if he ran fartlek, rather than straight distance: "Rather than doing mindless 20-milers, you vary the pace, which forces you to pay attention." Sue King, while training for the New York City Marathon, found she could concentrate more by running long runs alone so the conversation of friends did not distract her.

"The physical training your body does during the 18-week buildup to the marathon can all be washed away if the mind wanders," says Frank Walaitis, a 3:02 runner from Carpentersville, Illinois.

Rodgers believes concentration must begin before a race. He avoids warming up with others, preferring to focus on the upcoming race. He also believes that the clinics, dinners, and social events he often attended as part of sponsor commitments diminished his concentration.

Nevertheless, many runners are less interested in developing or maintaining their powers of concentration in order to run fast. They are more interested in keeping mind and body together long enough to finish!

Judith Henderson of Denver, Colorado, counts steps—almost for the entire length of the race. "If I count every left-foot plant," says Henderson, "it takes 440 left steps to run a mile. I keep the game up even through aid stations and brief conversations with other runners. It's like a mental metronome. In the final miles of the marathon, I keep my focus on just the numbers, and it's amazing how much this helps to keep moving you forward."

Tracy Musacchio of New York City works out math problems in her head: "It's 70 degrees out. What's that in Celsius? How high can I name prime numbers? What's 86 squared? It seems silly, but it works for me."

While training for a marathon, Lori Hauswirth of Merrill, Wisconsin, keeps herself moving with what might be considered personal threats. "If I'm having a bad run, I tell myself that if I stop to walk, I won't qualify for Boston," she says.

Autumn Evans of Melbourne Beach, Florida, uses a similar drill sergeant approach when it comes to the final miles: "I resort to telling myself, 'Suck it up, you weenie!' I don't want to disappoint myself by giving up or quitting."

Nicole Long of St. Louis used an omen to spur her to a Boston qualifying time. "I told myself around 19 miles that I'd qualify for Boston if I saw a beagle on the course. So I spent the next several miles looking for one. Luckily, I spotted a man with a beagle. Later I saw the same man and his beagle at the finish line. I thanked him for bringing it."

HOW TO FOCUS

It may be risky for a runner to depend on the supply of beagles in the crowd for success. Ultimately, learning to improve your attention span and ability to concentrate for longer periods may prove to be the best strategy. But how can you learn to concentrate? How do you focus your mind on the business at foot?

At least one study shows that the average runner can learn to think like the elite runner. Researcher Hein Helgo Schomer, PhD, of the University of Cape Town in South Africa, improved the concentration of a group of ten non-elite runners over a period of 5 weeks. Before they were coached, the runners used association (being tuned in to their bodies) only 45 percent of the time. By the fifth week under Schomer's instruction, they were associating 70 percent of the time while running, and their average training intensity also increased.

Think like the elite.

Learning to concentrate takes time. Each spring, once the snow melted, I used to head to the track for weekly interval training to try to regain speed lost after a winter of slow running. When I ran quarters, I knew that to run my fastest, I had to concentrate. Yet invariably I would get on the back stretch and my mind would wander and my pace would lag. Only after 5 or 6 weeks did my concentration improve to the point where I could keep my attention on running for a full quarter as well as during the interval of slow running between quarters. My track times then started to drop, convincing me that the improvement resulted from both stronger muscles and a stronger mind.

THE FINAL 6 MILES

Past 20 miles is when mental strategies become most important. Conversation between friends usually has ceased by then. It's gut-it-out and head for the finish line. During the final 6 miles, concentration often spells the difference between a good and bad race. Here are some suggestions from marathoners who have used mental strategies to achieve success.

Jim Fredericks, South Milwaukee, Wisconsin: "I think about where I would be on my home training course. Six miles to go is the Grant Park Golf Course. Four miles to go is South Milwaukee High School. It makes the remaining distance seem somewhat shorter when I put it in that perspective."

Melissa Vetricek, Tampa, Florida: "It's too overwhelming to think of how many miles remain. I think minutes. When my body wants to walk, I tell it, 'Run for just 8 more minutes.' That's about how long it takes to cover a mile. When those 8 minutes are up, I say, 'Eight minutes more.' Sometimes when I'm really hurting, I say, 'One more minute' or 'Just take 90 steps more.' I'll bargain with the devil when it comes to those last half dozen miles."

Colleen Gibbs, Carlsbad, California: "I use crazy ideas to counteract negative thoughts. Mick Jagger eating a banana on a unicycle worked one time. Just the distraction of conjuring up the visual pushed bad thoughts aside and killed a few of those last, long minutes."

Bob Winter, New Lenox, Illinois: "I dedicate each mile to someone, whether publicly or privately. Beginning with the next mile marker, I keep them in my thoughts. I use them for extra motivation, knowing that I'll have to report to them postrace about their mile."

Andrew Smith, Omaha, Nebraska: "I pick out a relatively close landmark and tell myself that I will run at least that far. Just before I arrive, I pick out another landmark farther down the road."

Barbara Mayer, Athens, Georgia: "I often dedicate marathons to a loved one or friend who has passed away. During the last few hundred yards of the 2001 Chicago Marathon (a month after September 11), I started to sing 'God Bless America' as loud as I could. Once I started, I couldn't stop because everybody was looking at me. I'm sure they all knew what was going through my mind."

I typically did 400-meter repeats (with a 400 jog in between) to prepare myself for track races. Marathoners might benefit from doing long repeats of a mile: 1600 meters, or four laps around a track. I even have done 2-mile repeats around a subdivision loop near my home. I say 2 miles, but I never measured the loop; I figured it was about 2 miles based on the time it took to run it. The loop might have been longer or shorter, but the confidence I got from nailing a "fast time" became one of my mind games.

I also found various forms of speedwork—tempo runs and fartlek in the woods and strides on the grass, in addition to intervals on the track—to be effective in improving my concentration. Sometimes I would head to the golf course several times a week to run a half dozen or more short sprints—not flat-out but close to the speed I reach in a track mile. I did these "strides" to loosen my muscles for other longer and tougher workouts. I would return from the golf course running much faster, with my mind totally focused.

Although sometimes I would have difficulty concentrating during track workouts, particularly on distance runs, I usually managed to get my act together for important races: Competition tended to focus my mind. It enabled me to achieve speeds in competition that were beyond my reach in training.

MIND AND BODY

How do you get mind and body in tune to run long distances faster? Here are several tips to help you block out mind drift.

Prepare yourself. Have a game plan for workouts and particularly for important races. Where are you going to run? How fast? How far? Against whom? Get yourself in a running frame of mind. Learn to relax. Following a regular warmup routine before running can get you into the mood to perform. Find a routine that works best for you—whether chanting a mantra or stretching—and stick with it.

> The ability to concentrate separates the merely good runners from the great ones.

Discover how your body works. While running fast, try to be aware of what the various parts of your body are doing. Can you discover what it feels like to run smoothly? If so, you may be able to duplicate that feeling on other occasions. Remember: Given equal physical skills, the ability to concentrate separates the merely good runners from the great ones.

Practice instant preplay and replay. If you can imagine before running how top runners run successfully—preplay—you're halfway to emulating them. Practice running mentally as well as physically. Try replay as well. When you run well, remember how you ran. Fix that image in your memory, adding it to your mental video library.

Head for the track. Running against the clock and attempting to match preset goals forces you to concentrate. Learning to adjust to the track's rhythm—running turns, for example—also helps, as do fartlek sessions and other forms of speedwork done on trails and on the road.

Plan days of maximum concentration. Not every workout needs to be fully focused, but select at least 1 day each week to practice concentration. Racing, particularly track or cross-country races, may help focus your mind.

Avoid race day distractions. Friends, traffic, or dogs (even beagles) can distract you from the act and art of running. Run solo when you can, to improve your concentration. If you want to succeed with your race plan, keep conversation to a minimum even if you are running with a friend.

Talk to yourself. Paul D. Thompson, MD, director of preventive cardiology at Hartford Hospital in Connecticut, believes runners need pep talks. "I talk to myself when I train," he says. "The year I ran best at Boston, I focused on what to tell myself during those last few miles, when it hurts." Thompson placed sixteenth at Boston one year by telling himself "Keep going" and "I'm a tough dude."

Landmark the course. What are the key points on the course you plan to race? Where are the hills? Where are the flats? What sections of the course will drain you, and what sections (such as by Wellesley College, where the women come out to cheer Boston marathoners) will give you strength? Do not wait until the course tour the day before the race to learn what you will be running.

Focus hardest when it counts most. If you find it difficult to concentrate during the full 26 miles of a marathon, save your focus for the miles when you need it the most. Kardong used to dissociate the first half of the race, then associate the second half.

Concentration cannot compensate for lack of training or basic ability, but it can help you maximize your potential.

23

Mile 27

Wait: Don't Stop Yet!

The most important mile of the marathon may be mile 27, the one you walk to the hotel. Shortly after finishing the Boston Marathon one year, I sat huddled on a bench in Copley Square, wrapped in an aluminum blanket, in one hand a soft drink and in the other a cup of frozen yogurt that I was too nauseated to eat. I cursed having stayed at a hotel whose distance from the finish line would require that I walk another mile—a 27th mile, so to speak—before I could end that day's marathon experience. Yet 15 minutes later, halfway to the hotel, frozen yogurt consumed, sipping a second soft drink, I felt my energy returning. I knew I would recover and eventually run 26 miles again.

That 27th mile is particularly important when it comes to speeding postmarathon recovery so that you can run and race again. Your actions during the first 5 seconds after crossing the line may be crucial to your recovery—as are the next 5 minutes, the next 5 hours, the next 5 days, and even the next 5 weeks. Postmarathon recovery is something many runners pay scant attention to. But by organizing your postrace plans as well as you do your prerace plans, you can recover faster and more comfortably and minimize future injuries.

DAMAGE CONTROL

"Runners need to take responsibility for the health of their muscles, not just how fast they go," warns Linda Jaros, a massage therapist from Dedham, Massachusetts, whose clients have included Bill Rodgers and Joan Benoit Samuelson. "Recovery has to become an integral part of their training."

Indeed, recovery may be the toughest skill for a marathon runner to master. How do you snap back after more than 26 hard miles on the road? Are fatigued and sore muscles inevitable, or are there strategies you can use to make marathon recovery not only faster but less painful? What secrets can we learn from both elite and ordinary marathoners that will allow a quick return to full training—and the next starting line? What do scientists suggest based on laboratory research, not only for the morning after, but also for the weeks after?

David L. Costill, PhD, of the Human Performance Laboratory at Ball State University in Muncie, Indiana, has researched, both in the lab and on the road, the damage marathons do to the body. In numerous studies, Dr. Costill has reviewed the postrace drinking, eating, and training habits of marathoners. His suggestions for recovery: Drink plenty of fluids, carbo-load after the race (as well as before), and don't start running again too soon.

> **Carbo-load after the race as well as before.**

"A lot of things happen to the body as a result of running the marathon," he adds. "You become overheated, dehydrated, and muscle depleted. Your hormonal milieu gets thrown out of whack, and you traumatize your muscles. You have to bide your time to get your body back in balance."

Jack H. Scaff, Jr., MD, founded the Honolulu Marathon and has supervised the Honolulu Marathon Clinic, a group that meets Sundays in Kapiolani Park to train for that marathon. After watching his group's recuperative efforts after the race one year, Dr. Scaff commented, "The runners felt so good about their achievement, they would bounce back too soon. The rate of injuries was exponential. We finally canceled the clinic for 3 months following the marathon to try to get the runners to take it easy."

Benji Durden of Boulder, Colorado, has observed the effects of marathon running on the body as a runner and as a coach of others, both fast and slow. Durden recalls running a 2:15 at Boston in 1978—cutting 4 minutes off his best time—then spraining an ankle the following week. "My body had not fully recovered," he notes. While conceding that total rest may be the best postmarathon prescription, Durden contends that runners may have conflicting psychological needs. "As a coach, I try to accept the best advice from the scientists and adapt it based on a combination of intuition and experience," he says.

KEEP MOVING

Want to recover as rapidly as possible following your next marathon? First, do not stop as soon as you cross the finish line. You may have no choice, particularly at major races where you will be prodded to jog and walk through the finish chute, after which you run a gauntlet that includes having various items pressed onto you: your medal, fluids and food, an aluminum blanket, and your gear brought from the starting line. Having accepted all this, you may need to walk what seems an unconscionably long distance to be greeted by friends and family.

This is not all bad.

Whether prodded or not, you need to keep moving to allow your stressed system a chance to gradually attain a steady state and also to avoid what Dr. Scaff calls the postrace collapse phenomenon. This, he says, is when "a runner looks good coming across the finish line, sits down too soon, then 20 minutes later must be taken to the first aid tent with heatstroke or cramps." Blood pressure can drop too quickly, sometimes with disastrous results. "Walking around a bit seems to prevent this from happening," says Dr. Scaff.

How much you walk depends on your condition at the end of the race. "If your body is telling you to collapse in a heap, walking around is not easy," says Dr. Costill. "But continuing to move for a while will maintain your circulation, keeping the blood pumping through the muscles. This should aid short-term recovery."

DEAD MEN WALKING

Most runners concede that walking a mile or two after finishing a marathon probably promotes quick recovery. Forcing yourself to do so, however, is not always easy—unless you get lost, as did Matt Ferrara of Troy, New York, after the Buffalo Marathon. Despite staying only one block from the finish line, Ferrara somehow missed his hotel and walked nearly a mile before realizing it. "When I finally got back to the hotel," he recalls, "I was feeling good enough to drive to Niagara Falls for some sightseeing."

"Walking is a great way to cool down," says Michele Keane of Atlanta, Georgia. "After the Chicago Marathon one year, I spent the rest of the afternoon walking and shopping up and down Michigan Avenue. It was great to have salesclerks and other shoppers ask me how I did, since I wore my medal proudly."

Paula Sue Russell of Findlay, Ohio, recalls finishing her first marathon with friends in Chicago: "We walked through the recovery area, gathering bagels, yogurt, water, and Gatorade. I was fine until we got to the Bud beer area. Everyone sat down on the ground to drink their beer. By the time I got my stiff body down, everyone was finished and getting up to leave."

Warning: Do not take the advice to keep moving to extremes. Many compulsive runners feel the need to "cool down" by jogging a mile or two, even after a marathon. Although this may make sense following a 10K race, it is not wise after a 42.2K race. No scientific studies have shown any benefits from postrace running. You simply increase your chance of injury by continuing to run.

DRINK UP

As long as you are walking, head in the direction of the tables with fluids. All the experts—scientists and experienced marathoners alike—recommend that you begin an immediate and continuing effort to replace the several liters of liquid your system has lost during 26 miles on the road. Grab the first cup of liquid thrust into your hand and start sipping at once, no matter how nauseated you feel.

Dr. Scaff recommends sipping at the rate of ½ ounce a minute. And while going about other recuperative activities for the next several hours, keep a drink in your hand and continue drinking.

Like most experts, Dr. Costill emphasizes that human thirst is not an accurate gauge of dehydration. "Drink more than you desire," he advises.

If the first cup thrust into your hand is water, accept it thankfully, but look for the table where they have drinks with at least some dilute form of sugar, whether in a so-called replacement drink (such as Gatorade), a soft drink, or a fruit drink. Your primary need is to replace fluids, but you have also depleted your muscles of glycogen and need to replace that as well. "Try to get your blood sugar back to normal as quickly as possible," says Durden. The best time for glycogen replacement, according to research by Edward F. Coyle, PhD, of the department of kinesiology at the University of Texas at Austin, is during the first 2 hours after the race. "The muscles absorb glycogen like a sponge," he says. "Four and 6 hours after the race, the absorption rate starts to decline." Nutritionists may argue that fruit drinks (because they contain vitamins and minerals) are superior to sugar drinks—and this certainly is true—but Dr. Costill claims that when it comes to glycogen replacement, the body does not know the difference between one sugar and another.

Two postmarathon drinks to avoid: diet soft drinks because they provide no glucose boost (having just burned approximately 2,600 calories, you should not focus on calorie restriction) and alcoholic beverages because they serve as a diuretic. That postrace beer may taste good, but it will eventually have a negative effect on fluid balance. If you drink a beer, do so only after you already have ingested twice the volume of other fluids. Another good choice for postrace nutrition is an energy bar, but Liz Applegate, PhD, a professor at the University of California at Davis and author of *Eat Smart, Play Hard*, suggests that you carefully read the labels before deciding which energy bar to ingest prerace and which to save for postrace. "Not all energy bars have the same purpose," warns Dr. Applegate. "Before the race, you want a bar that is almost entirely carbohydrates. But after the race, your choice should be a bar with some protein added, which will promote recovery."

You need to keep moving.

OFF YOUR FEET

After spending the first 5 to 10 minutes walking around and obtaining something to drink, get off your feet. Listen to your body. "Do what it tells you to do," says Dr. Costill. "Get horizontal." Pick a comfortable spot, preferably in the shade, and elevate your feet, easing the flow of blood to the heart. Dr. Costill speculates that some of the muscle soreness and stiffness experienced immediately after a race may be related to edema, swelling caused by the intramuscular pressure of accumulated fluids in the lower legs. "Elevating the legs may speed recovery," he says.

You can assist your recovery with gentle self-massage. But do not knead. Stroke your leg muscles gently toward the heart. Massage with ice to reduce the swelling. Hosing your legs with cold water is another option. An ice bath may be even better.

Bill Rodgers, winner of the Boston and New York City Marathons four times each, likes to do some postrace stretching while lying down. If you choose to do the same, do not stretch excessively. Your muscles most likely are stiff and damaged; you do not want to traumatize them further.

Some experts even question the value of stretching. A study at the University of Texas at Tyler indicated that static stretching failed to prevent muscle soreness later. Researchers Katherine C. Buroker and James A. Schwane, PhD, concede that stretching helps maintain flexibility, but they say that stretching immediately after strenuous exercise may be the wrong time for it.

Avoid hot baths.

When Dr. Scaff surveyed members of his Honolulu Marathon Clinic, he discovered that those who stretched most also had the most injuries. Or maybe after becoming injured, they began a stretching routine. Scientists remain divided on the value of stretching, so your best bet is to keep any stretching short and simple after a marathon.

While resting, continue to sip fluids, your primary recovery strategy. (Using a bent straw makes it easier to drink while horizontal.) To guarantee a supply, place a bottle of your favorite postrace drink in the bag you plan to check. If you do not have to use it, no problem. Better to have too much fluid available than too little.

BEGIN TO REFUEL

Your immediate concern after the race may have been fluid replacement, but within an hour after finishing, you should begin shifting to more solid foods. This may be particularly important if sugar from replacement drinks makes you feel ill, as food can slow down sugar absorption to help prevent the nausea. Ken Young, a top trail runner and Pikes Peak Marathon winner from Northern California, liked to eat saltines to help settle his stomach. Fruit is a good start, particularly bananas, because they are easy to digest and provide a good way to replace lost potassium. Do not become obsessed with instant mineral replacement, however. Eating several well-balanced meals within the next 24 hours will take care of electrolytes lost through sweating.

Research by Dr. Coyle indicates that 1 gram of carbohydrate per kilogram of body weight per hour is necessary for the most efficient glycogen replacement. That translates to 2 calories per pound, or 300 calories for a 150-pound runner. Sports dietitian Nancy Clark suggests that a marathoner drink a glass of orange juice and eat one banana and a cup of yogurt the first hour, then repeat that the second hour.

As a practical matter, I'll grab anything handy, particularly those chocolate chip cookies at the end of the table. Immediately after a marathon, I am like a shark feeding. Anything in close range of my mouth gets consumed.

MASSAGE

Many major marathons provide massage tents with teams of trained massage therapists ready to give a soothing rubdown. Early finishers sometimes head straight to that tent to beat the crowd, but it is preferable to wait 45 minutes so you can give yourself time to rehydrate and cool down. And do not allow therapists to poke and probe your muscles as vigorously as they might during a regular session. The best postmarathon massage, according to therapist Rich Phaigh of Eugene, Oregon, begins with the lower back and the buttocks to relax those muscles and get intramuscular fluids flowing, then works gently on the legs with long, flowing motions toward the heart. If the massage hurts, ask the therapist to be gentler; if it still hurts, thank the therapist graciously and get off the table.

For those athletes with a regular massage therapist, the best time for a massage is 24 to 48 hours after the race, the time when muscle soreness usually peaks. In preparing for marathons, I schedule appointments with my regular massage therapist the afternoon before the race and 2 days after. When running in a different city—or a different country—I try to locate a massage therapist by networking with other runners. It is amazing how the Internet has made it easier to do this.

Avoid hot baths or showers, which may increase inflammation and unnecessarily elevate your body temperature. That bubbling whirlpool back at the motel may look inviting, but leave it to the kids. Opt for a cool shower. "Getting your body temperature back down will help you recover faster," says Dr. Costill.

Amanda Musacchio, one of my cousins from Wheaton, Illinois, strongly believes in ice baths. She has converted many runners into adopting this admittedly scary practice. You fill your bathtub with cold water, then add ice cubes to drop the temperature even further before sliding gently into the water. "Ice baths sound painful," says Musacchio, "but they really speed recovery by reducing swelling." After long runs I often chill my legs similarly, wading into either Lake Michigan or the Atlantic Ocean, depending on whether I am at home in Indiana or in Florida.

Aspirin and anti-inflammatories should be avoided. Although their use seemingly should reduce the pain of sore muscles, their use also prolongs the time required to repair damage.

HANGING OUT

Most marathoners do not want to abandon the scene of battle too rapidly. Admittedly, part of the enjoyment of marathoning is hanging around to see old friends and rivals, cheering their finishes, and swapping stories about the miles just covered. Do not deny yourself the opportunity to wallow awhile in the joy of your accomplishment, regardless of the commonsense advice I have just offered you.

But after you have showered, jump into bed. Even if you have difficulty sleeping, at least rest for 1 to 2 hours. Then get up: It's time for more food.

Three to 4 hours after finishing, sit down to a full meal. Dr. Costill claims that carbohydrates should still be the food of choice. "Nutritionally, your first meal after the marathon should resemble your last meal before," he says. Sound advice, although many marathoners rebel against having to look at one more plate of pasta and instead indulge a sudden craving for protein.

"I'm not afraid to eat a hamburger after a marathon," says Doug Kurtis. "It almost feels like a reward." Bill Rodgers recalls going to a restaurant one year after placing third in the Boston Marathon and eating a hamburger, followed by a hot fudge sundae. He also fondly recalls family victory celebrations at his running store with picnic lunches of chicken sandwiches supplied by his mother.

But remember that spaghetti is not the only source of carbohydrates. "Even high-carbohydrate diets have some protein," says Clark. "Your body needs to rebuild protein, so have your chicken or steak or fish, but start with some minestrone soup. Add some extra potatoes, rolls, and juice. The secret in anything you eat is moderation. Don't focus on the meat; focus on the carbohydrates that can accompany the meat."

TIME OUT

Once home, too many marathoners make the mistake of resuming training too soon. They may fear getting out of shape or feel that some easy jogging will help speed their recovery. Research by Dr. Costill suggests the opposite: that recovery is speeded and conditioning not affected if you do nothing for 7 to 10 days after the race.

Durden thinks it is all right to resume easy running by the fourth day. The recovery programs available on my website reflect that same philosophy. Durden warns against the cross-training used by some recuperating marathoners. "When I say rest, I mean rest," he says. "Not weightlifting. Not Exercycling. Not swimming. Not walking. You rest! I've worked with a few athletes who thought 'rest' meant everything except 'run.'"

Moving in the pool is another matter. It may comfort the muscles if you immerse yourself in water and use gentle, nonaerobic movements to stretch and relax your arms and legs. But do not start doing laps, because you will simply delay recovery by burning more glycogen. (It may be a good idea to go back and review the pool running chapter on page 168.)

RETURN SLOWLY

Once you return to running, do not run too hard or too fast too soon. Bill Rodgers took his time coming back after marathons. "Slowly, over a period of weeks, I'd build back to regular mileage. I'd stick with once-a-day training for a while. No speed or long runs for at least 2 or 3 weeks."

Particularly after a good performance, runners need to resist the urge to come back too soon under the theory that more work may mean still better times. "You end up pushing yourself too hard," warns Durden. "You may get away with it for 4 to 6 weeks; then you collapse, get injured, get sick, or feel stale and overtrained. The period immediately after a good marathon is when you need to be especially cautious about your training." Russell H. Pate, PhD, chairman of the department of exercise science at the University of South Carolina in Columbia, developed a 2-week recovery method through trial and error. "I'd have very minimal activity for 2 to 3 days after the race; still modest running for the remainder of the 1st week; then, over the 2nd week, gradually build to near my normal training loads. By the 3rd week, I'd be ready to run hard again." But on one occasion when he felt good after 3 days and resumed heavy training too quickly, 3 weeks later he had a breakdown, featuring minor injuries and fatigue. "I learned the hard way to put the brakes on," Dr. Pate recalls.

> **"When I say rest, I mean rest."**

"Studies now show you do indeed damage the muscle, creating micro-trauma in muscle fibers, with activities like marathon running," he says. "No one knows what we do to the connective tissue and skeleton, but I suspect there's trauma there also. Since scientists do not yet know precisely how much time is needed for such trauma to be reversed, it's smart for runners to give themselves plenty of time with minimal running to let that healing process occur."

None of the experts—neither scientists nor coaches nor experienced road runners—can offer an exact formula for marathon recovery. Too many factors are involved, from the condition of the runner going into the race to the conditions of the race itself. Hilly courses, particularly those with downhills near the end, such as Boston, do more muscle damage than flat courses. Extremes of heat or cold slow the recovery process. And runners who start out too fast and crash seem to have more difficulty recovering than do those who run an even pace.

"Nature takes care of us," concedes Dr. Costill. "Time heals most of the damage done in the marathon." Through careful attention to the 27th mile, most of us will be back on the road again, looking forward to our next trip to the starting line.

POSTMARATHON SYNDROME

Runners crossing the finish line of a marathon do so with a combination of exhaustion and exultation. For many, it is the most exciting moment in their lives; it may also be among the most painful. Yet runners raise their arms in victory—even though twenty thousand or more others may have finished in front of them.

A day later, after the shining medal hanging from its colorful ribbon has been placed in a drawer, the same runners must face

(continued)

the question of what to do next. They encounter the postmarathon blues.

"We focus our lives on this one event for 5 months—and then it's done," reflects Autumn Evans of Melbourne Beach, Florida. "Now what?"

For the immediate several weeks, runners such as Evans can focus on repairing their bodies. On my website, I feature a postmarathon training schedule that involves 5 weeks of rest and easy running. That takes care of the body, but what about the mind?

One way to cope with postmarathon blues is to pick a new goal. Maybe it is another marathon. Maybe it is a faster time. Setting a PR or qualifying for the Boston Marathon presents a challenge to many. Your goal need not be another 26-miler. Other runners add swimming and cycling to their fitness routine and point to a triathlon.

And your next goal does not need to be running-related. One friend of mine decided in her midforties to learn to play the violin. Would taking a course in computer science improve your business skills? How about reconnecting with those people in your life whom you abandoned temporarily while doing 4-hour runs as part of your marathon buildup?

"I didn't train properly before my first marathon," confesses Cherie Robideaux of Hailey, Idaho. "My knees hurt so badly, I swore I'd never run again. I got over those postmarathon blues, and I'm already looking forward to my next marathon."

24

BQ

Boston Remains the Ultimate Goal
for Many Runners

One huge standard of achievement is running fast enough to qualify for the Boston Marathon, the granddaddy of American marathons. For three-quarters of a century, the Boston Marathon accepted almost anyone who showed up at Hopkinton Gym on race day with a $1 entry fee in hand. You did not yet need to offer proof that you had run a previous marathon in a qualifying time, what today is known as a BQ (Boston qualifier). Following Amateur Athletic Union rules then in place, you would submit to a physical exam to ensure that you would not die of a heart attack and embarrass the organizers, but qualify for the race? No need. In the early years, us marathoners were few and far between. Until 1970, the largest field at the Boston Athletic Association Marathon (its official name) had been 285 runners in 1928.

Then in the 1960s, a seismic shift occurred. Running suddenly became popular as health-conscious baby boomers edged into middle age. For at least some, the Boston Marathon became a goal akin to the ascent of Mount Everest. In 1960, according to Tom Derderian's history, *Boston*

Marathon, only 156 started the race. A decade later in 1970, that number skyrocketed to 1,011, with 678 finishing under 4 hours.

I accept some of the blame (or credit) for the increase. In 1963, I wrote an article for *Sports Illustrated* titled "On the Run from Dogs and People," focused on the Boston Marathon. Entries jumped from 285 that year to a record 369 the following year, and it seemed like several dozen individuals introduced themselves to me in the Hopkinton Gym saying they had started running (with Boston their goal) after reading my article. In truth, the bestselling book *Aerobics* by Kenneth L. Cooper, MD, and the gold medal won by American Frank Shorter at the 1972 Olympic Games did more to ignite the running boom, but long-distance running with Boston as its kingpin suddenly had become a mainstream activity.

The Boston Marathon at that time was organized part time by two individuals. Will Cloney was a sportswriter. Jock Semple was a trainer for the Boston Bruins and the Boston Celtics. They greeted the burgeoning number of marathoners with panic, fearing that the narrow roads between suburban Hopkinton and downtown Boston could not support more than 1,000 runners. So they imposed a qualifying time of 4 hours to limit the field to less than 1,000 runners.

Boston's qualifying requirement merely spurred runners to train harder. Boston became the standard for marathon excellence. By qualifying for the Boston Marathon, runners achieved status among their peers. It earned you bragging rights to be able to say nonchalantly that you had "qualified for Boston." Boston's numbers continued to increase because once a runner qualified, it seemed almost obligatory to go to Boston to run. So the organizers lowered the standard from 4:00 to 3:30 to 3:00, until by the mid-1980s, if you were a male under 40, you had to run 2:50 to qualify.

That 2:50 standard was too tough. Four hours is a reasonable time for a runner of average ability who is willing to train hard, but to run the course more than an hour faster requires a certain natural ability. To get into the Boston Marathon, you needed to combine talent and training. Eventually, Boston relaxed its standards to 3:10 for the fastest age group

(18 to 34), with a sliding scale of slower times in other categories, depending on age and sex. After the 2011 race filled in only 8 hours 3 minutes, the BAA toughened its standards and changed its registration procedures.

Currently, Boston limits its field to approximately 30,000 entrants, with 80 percent of them "qualified" runners and the rest runners who secure their starting-line positions by raising money for various charities. In 2019, charity runners raised $38.7 million. For the 2020 Boston Marathon, the qualifying standards for different age groups began at 3:00 for men ages 18 to 34 and 3:30 for women ages 18 to 34. The BQ standards often change from year to year. Current standards can be found on the BAA website: www.baa.org. How do you secure a BQ? What training program guarantees you a spot on the starting line? Let me be honest with you. Training programs, mine and those offered by other coaches, do *not* carry a guarantee. Each runner succeeds or fails by how well he or she trains and, yes, a certain level of talent is required. Nevertheless, you can improve your BQ chances if you do the following:

1. Think far, far ahead. Most of my marathon training programs last 18 weeks, but that may not be enough time. Unless you have enormous talent (and some folk do), you may need a year or two or more to gradually become a better (and smarter) runner, allowing you to secure a BQ. In my book *Hal Higdon's How to Train*, I featured a program designed by Olympian Benji Durden that lasted 84 weeks and featured two half marathons and two marathons. In terms of time, Benji got it right. Exercise patience, and it may take a failure or two before you experience success.

2. Pick your qualifying marathon carefully. Most marathons provide life-changing experiences, but not all are equal when it comes to providing a qualifying opportunity. Hills or heat or both may rise to confound you, so look for races where the course is flat (or even downhill) and the weather is lovely more often than not. (See the accompanying sidebar for the marathons that produce the most Boston qualifiers.)

3. Get serious, and I mean really serious. You love running 5Ks and 10Ks, and there's that fun half marathon that you do every year. Okay, racing is fun, but too much racing can drain psychic as much as physical energy. If you want that BQ, Boston must become a singular goal, not one of many goals.

4. Pickup basketball games are not cross-training. Neither is soccer. Neither is volleyball. And although cycling and swimming do qualify as cross-training, too much of those activities will not make you a better runner. If you get injured participating in other sports (cross-training or not), kiss that BQ attempt goodbye.

5. Some nonrunning activities are permitted. If achieving that BQ totally dominates your life, maybe you need to relax. Planning a family vacation? Reread tip #1: *Think far, far ahead.* If you have planned well, you can modify your training schedule to allow necessary downtime. All my marathon training programs have step-back weeks. And if you're on a cruise, the biggest ships feature running tracks on the top deck.

6. Watch what you eat. Run past that cruise ship buffet. A lot of runners assume that as long as they run a lot of miles, they can eat whatever they want. Prime rib? Sounds great. Burgers right off the grill? What could be better? But maybe it is time to rethink your nutritional habits. Definitely avoid any weight-loss diets that might push you into a caloric deficit. Going on a crash diet to shed a few pounds should never be part of any BQ strategy.

7. The last few days are critical. Think of your comfort. Travel is not cheap—neither are airfares nor hotel rooms—but you invested a great deal of time and effort in your training. Raid the penny jar so you can afford to arrive in town a day early. A massage that final week might provide just the edge of prerace relaxation you need.

8. Don't overlook your hometown. Considering all of the above, your hometown marathon may not be as "fast" as the ten listed here, but sleeping in your own bed may be worth an extra minute or two off your time. Being in a race where family and friends not only can cheer you but also can hand you something to drink or eat has got to be worth a few more seconds off the clock, and those few seconds may get you your Boston qualifier.

FINDING YOUR BQ

Which marathons produce the most Boston qualifiers? Not surprisingly, Boston leads the list, with many in its field requalifying for the next year's race. Size allows Chicago (45,000) and New York (53,000) to provide large numbers of BQ runners, Chicago having a flatter course than New York. Among other top-ten BQ races, several have downhill courses, but you need to train specifically to run downhill or your quad muscles will be mush before you reach 20. If the wind is blowing from the wrong direction on a point-to-point course, that may undo you. Add in the variability of weather. There are no guarantees when you step to the starting line of a marathon, but under most conditions, good training will allow you to achieve success.

1. Boston Marathon

2. Chicago Marathon

3. New York City Marathon

4. California International Marathon (Sacramento)

5. Philadelphia Marathon

6. Erie Marathon (PA)

7. Mountains 2 Beach Marathon (Ventura, CA)

8. Mount Charleston Marathon (Las Vegas, NV)

9. Berlin Marathon

10. Indianapolis Monumental Marathon

IT'S TIME TO RUN BOSTON

Now that you've qualified, how do you train for what is almost guaranteed to be a momentous experience? Welcome to Boston Bound. This 13-week program is aimed at those already qualified for Boston, not for those hoping to achieve a BQ. It starts in January, soon after the holidays, 13 weeks out. Long runs alternate between minutes and miles. Be aware that a 3/1 long run is easy the first three-quarters of the distance, then harder the final one-quarter. Hill training is necessary if you want to hit Heartbreak Hill in cruise control. Also, some of your hill training should include downhill repeats. This is not an easy program, but getting a BQ is not easy. If you are well-trained enough to include a BQ on your curriculum vitae it should not scare you.

A couple of warnings: It is not so much that the Boston Marathon has a difficult course (Heartbreak Hill is not that high), but it is a different course. Very few runners score PRs in their first Boston attempts. It took me five attempts to learn how to run Boston, but now I get to pass on what I learned to you. Get it right, training for Boston and racing at Boston, and you can join the best long-distance runners in the world.

Boston Bound

Week	Mon	Tue	Wed	Thu	Fri	Sat	Sun
1	3-mile run easy	3 × hill, 1 down	3-mile run easy	5-mile tempo	Rest	6-mile pace	1:20, 3/1
2	4-mile run easy	4 × 800, 400 jog	4-mile run easy	7-mile tempo	Rest	7-mile pace	14-mile run easy
3	4-mile run easy	4 × hill, 1 down	4-mile run easy	7-mile run easy	Rest	7-mile easy	1:30, 3/1
4	4-mile run easy	5 × 800, 400 jog	4-mile run easy	5-mile run easy	Rest	7-mile pace	16-mile run easy
5	4-mile run easy	5 × hill, 2 down	4-mile run easy	8-mile tempo	Rest	5K race	1:40, 3/1
6	5-mile run easy	6 × 800, 400 jog	5-mile run easy	8-mile run easy	Rest	8-mile pace	18-mile run easy
7	5-mile run easy	6 × hill, 2 down	5-mile run easy	5-mile tempo	Rest	10K race	1:50, 3/1
8	5-mile run easy	7 × 800, 400 jog	5-mile run easy	8-mile run easy	Rest	5-mile run easy	20-mile run easy
9	5-mile run easy	7 × hill, 3 down	5-mile run easy	5-mile run easy	Rest	Half marathon	2:00, 3/1
10	5-mile run easy	8 × 800, 400 jog	5-mile run easy	8-mile run easy	Rest	5-mile pace	20-mile run easy
11	5-mile run easy	8 × hill, 3 down	5-mile run easy	6-mile tempo	Rest	4-mile pace	12-mile run easy
12	5-mile run easy	4 × 800, 400 jog	5-mile run easy	4-mile tempo	Rest	Rest	2-mile run easy
13	Boston						

PROGRAMS

To Reach Your Goals, Train Smart

Simplicity. That is a word that I like to associate with all of my programs: those that follow and the many more available online. And *simplicity* is not a word or concept that I chose; over the years many runners have approached me at races and expos to say what they liked most about my training programs was their simplicity. They're easy to understand and to follow.

For example, skip ahead a few pages in this chapter, and look at Marathon Novice 1: Monday, *Rest.* Tuesday, *Run.* Wednesday, *Run a little longer.* Thursday, *Run.* Friday, *Rest.* Saturday, *Run still longer.* Sunday, *Cross train.* Add a mile or two each week, and you arrive at the marathon after 18 weeks of effort fully trained and ready to fly. Doesn't get much simpler than that.

Life gets slightly more complex as you move from the novice programs through the intermediate programs to the advanced programs. But runners who start at Novice 1 and end at Advanced 2 learn while doing: Keep it simple, don't overtrain, and success is guaranteed.

More than half a million runners have trained for marathons using the programs featured here and in the previous four editions of this book. Here are my most popular programs for both the marathon and the half marathon, which increasingly has become a good "starter" event for runners who hope to leapfrog from 13.1 to 26.2.

HALF MARATHON: NOVICE 1

The Novice 1 half marathon program is a good place to begin. This is one of my easiest programs because of the relatively low mileage and the gentle ramp upward. Can you handle 4 miles running and/or walking? The workouts in Week 1 certainly are doable, even for beginners. Monday and Friday are rest days. Short runs are featured midweek with cross-training (bike, swim, walk) as a variation. Saturday is a cross-training day—30 to 60 minutes—a prelude to the long run on Sunday, which peaks at 10 miles in Week 11. Consider doing a 5K or 10K en route to your goal to get a feel for the racing experience.

Week	Mon	Tue	Wed	Thu	Fri	Sat	Sun
1	Rest	3-mile run	2-mile run or cross	3-mile run	Rest	30-min cross	4-mile run
2	Rest	3-mile run	2-mile run or cross	3-mile run	Rest	30-min cross	4-mile run
3	Rest	3.5-mile run	2-mile run or cross	3.5-mile run	Rest	40-min cross	5-mile run
4	Rest	3.5-mile run	2-mile run or cross	3.5-mile run	Rest	40-min cross	5-mile run
5	Rest	4-mile run	2-mile run or cross	4-mile run	Rest	40-min cross	6-mile run
6	Rest	4-mile run	2-mile run or cross	4-mile run	Rest or easy run	Rest	5K race
7	Rest	4.5-mile run	3-mile run or cross	4.5-mile run	Rest	50-min cross	7-mile run
8	Rest	4.5-mile run	3-mile run or cross	4.5-mile run	Rest	50-min cross	8-mile run
9	Rest	5-mile run	3-mile run or cross	5-mile run	Rest or easy run	Rest	10K race
10	Rest	5-mile run	3-mile run or cross	5-mile run	Rest	60-min cross	9-mile run
11	Rest	5-mile run	3-mile run or cross	5-mile run	Rest	60-min cross	10-mile run
12	Rest	4-mile run	3-mile run or cross	2-mile run	Rest	Rest	Half marathon

HALF MARATHON: NOVICE 2

The half marathon Novice 2 program provides only a slight step upward: a few more miles here, a few more miles there, but pretty much the same pattern as Novice 1. This program was designed for those who have been running more than a few months, individuals who have been accustomed to runs of a half-dozen miles or more. But it is also popular with experienced runners who have run half marathons before and do not want to overtrain before their next one. You don't necessarily have to take the leap between novice to intermediate.

Week	Mon	Tue	Wed	Thu	Fri	Sat	Sun
1	Rest	3-mile run	3-mile run	3-mile run	Rest	4-mile run	60-min cross
2	Rest	3-mile run	3-mile pace	3-mile run	Rest	5-mile run	60-min cross
3	Rest	3-mile run	4-mile run	3-mile run	Rest	6-mile run	60-min cross
4	Rest	3-mile run	4-mile pace	3-mile run	Rest	7-mile run	60-min cross
5	Rest	3-mile run	4-mile run	3-mile run	Rest	8-mile run	60-min cross
6	Rest	3-mile run	4-mile pace	3-mile run	Rest	5K race	60-min cross
7	Rest	3-mile run	5-mile run	3-mile run	Rest	9-mile run	60-min cross
8	Rest	3-mile run	5-mile pace	3-mile run	Rest	10-mile run	60-min cross
9	Rest	3-mile run	5-mile run	3-mile run	Rest	10K race	60-min cross
10	Rest	3-mile run	5-mile pace	3-mile run	Rest	11-mile run	60-min cross
11	Rest	3-mile run	5-mile run	3-mile run	Rest	12-mile run	60-min cross
12	Rest	3-mile run	2-mile pace	2-mile run	Rest	Rest	Half mara-thon

HALF MARATHON: INTERMEDIATE 1

Moving from the novice to the intermediate programs, you encounter a greater degree of difficulty. In Intermediate 1, I steal a day of rest from you on Mondays and suggest you cross-train. Tuesdays and Thursdays are twins, easy running. Wednesday runs are somewhat longer with several days featuring pace runs, workouts where you run at your half marathon pace, to learn that pace. Friday rest before a tough weekend with a few more pace runs and a long run schedule that takes you up to 12 miles just before your 13.1-mile race.

Week	Mon	Tue	Wed	Thu	Fri	Sat	Sun
1	30-min cross	3-mile run	4-mile run	3-mile run	Rest	3-mile run	4-mile run
2	30-min cross	3-mile run	4-mile pace	3-mile run	Rest	3-mile pace	5-mile run
3	40-min cross	3.5-mile run	5-mile run	3.5-mile run	Rest	Rest	6-mile run
4	40-min cross	3.5-mile run	5-mile pace	3.5-mile run	Rest	3-mile run	7-mile run
5	40-min cross	4-mile run	6-mile run	4-mile run	Rest	3-mile pace	8-mile run
6	50-min cross	4-mile run	6-mile pace	4-mile run	Rest or easy run	Rest	5K race
7	Rest	4.5-mile run	7-mile run	4.5-mile run	Rest	4-mile pace	9-mile run
8	50-min cross	4.5-mile run	7-mile pace	4.5-mile run	Rest	5-mile pace	10-mile run
9	60-min cross	5-mile run	8-mile run	5-mile run	Rest or easy run	Rest	10K race
10	Rest	5-mile run	8-mile pace	5-mile run	Rest	5-mile pace	11-mile run
11	60-min cross	5-mile run	6-mile run	4-mile run	Rest	3-mile pace	12-mile run
12	Rest	4-mile run	4-mile pace	2-mile run	Rest	Rest	Half mara-thon

HALF MARATHON: INTERMEDIATE 2

I like to think of Intermediate 1 as an endurance-based program. Nothing fast or fancy. Just go out and run some more miles than you did in the novice programs. Intermediate 2 features speedwork on Wednesdays, alternating between interval running at the track and tempo runs, possibly in the woods. (A tempo run is where you start slow, gradually accelerate to near 10K pace, hold, then decelerate to the slow pace at which you began.)

Week	Mon	Tue	Wed	Thu	Fri	Sat	Sun
1	30-min cross	3-mile run	5 × 400 5K pace	3-mile run	Rest	3-mile run	5-mile run
2	30-min cross	3-mile run	30-min tempo	3-mile run	Rest	3-mile pace	6-mile run
3	40-min cross	3.5-mile run	6 × 400 5K pace	3-mile run	Rest	Rest	5K race
4	40-min cross	3.5-mile run	35-min tempo	3-mile run	Rest	3-mile run	7-mile run
5	40-min cross	4-mile run	7 × 400 5K pace	3-mile run	Rest	3-mile pace	8-mile run
6	50-min cross	4-mile run	40-min tempo	3-mile run	Rest or easy run	Rest	10K race
7	Rest	4.5-mile run	8 × 400 5K pace	3-mile run	Rest	4-mile pace	9-mile run
8	50-min cross	4.5-mile run	40-min tempo	3-mile run	Rest	5-mile pace	10-mile run
9	60-min cross	5-mile run	9 × 400 5K pace	3-mile run	Rest or easy run	Rest	15K race
10	Rest	5-mile run	45-min tempo	3-mile run	Rest	5-mile pace	11-mile run
11	60-min cross	5-mile run	10 × 400 5K pace	3-mile run	Rest	3-mile pace	12-mile run
12	Rest	4-mile run	30-min tempo	2-mile run	Rest	Rest	Half marathon

HALF MARATHON: ADVANCED

Advanced Half Marathon is not for beginners. It will challenge you with speedwork on Tuesday, fast tempo runs on Thursday, some pace runs on Saturday, and long runs that lengthen a mile each week. In interval training you run a fast lap or two around the track, then jog or walk during the interval between to recover. Then repeat. Hill workouts are similar: Substitute a hill and run it with the same degree of difficulty as you do the track repeats. For the final week leading into the race, I consider 1 week sufficient taper for a half marathon, rather than the 3-week taper for marathons.

Week	Mon	Tue	Wed	Thu	Fri	Sat	Sun
1	3-mile run	6 × hill	3-mile run	40-min tempo	Rest	3-mile run	90-min run (3/1)
2	3-mile run	7 × 400 5K pace	3-mile run	45-min tempo	Rest	3-mile pace	90-min run
3	3-mile run	7 × hill	3-mile run	30-min tempo	Rest or easy run	Rest	5K race
4	3-mile run	8 × 400 5K pace	3-mile run	40-min tempo	Rest	3-mile run	90-min run (3/1)
5	3-mile run	8 × hill	3-mile run	45-min tempo	Rest	3-mile pace	90-min run
6	3-mile run	8 × 400 5K pace	3-mile run	30-min tempo	Rest or easy run	Rest	10K race
7	3-mile run	4 × 800 5K pace	3-mile run	45-min tempo	Rest	4-mile pace	1:45 run (3/1)
8	3-mile run	3 × 1600 race pace	3-mile run	50-min tempo	Rest	5-mile pace	1:45 run
9	3-mile run	5 × 800 10K pace	3-mile run	30-min tempo	Rest or easy run	Rest	15K race
10	3-mile run	4 × 1600 race pace	3-mile run	55-min tempo	Rest	5-mile pace	2:00 run (3/1)
11	3-mile run	6 × 800 10K pace	3-mile run	60-min tempo	Rest	3-mile pace	2:00 run
12	3-mile run	6 × 400 5K pace	2-mile run	30-min tempo	Rest	Rest	Half marathon

MARATHON: NOVICE 1

Shift your sights upward to the full marathon. Let's begin with Novice 1, my most popular program. The key to Novice 1 is the long run on Saturday: 6 miles in Week 1, progressing to 20 miles in the climactic Week 15.

Week	Mon	Tue	Wed	Thu	Fri	Sat	Sun
1	Rest	3-mile run	3-mile run	3-mile run	Rest	6-mile run	60-min cross
2	Rest	3-mile run	3-mile run	3-mile run	Rest	7-mile run	60-min cross
3	Rest	3-mile run	4-mile run	3-mile run	Rest	5-mile run	60-min cross
4	Rest	3-mile run	4-mile run	3-mile run	Rest	9-mile run	60-min cross
5	Rest	3-mile run	5-mile run	3-mile run	Rest	10-mile run	60-min cross
6	Rest	3-mile run	5-mile run	3-mile run	Rest	7-mile run	60-min cross
7	Rest	3-mile run	6-mile run	3-mile run	Rest	12-mile run	60-min cross
8	Rest	3-mile run	6-mile run	3-mile run	Rest	Rest	Half marathon
9	Rest	3-mile run	7-mile run	4-mile run	Rest	10-mile run	60-min cross
10	Rest	3-mile run	7-mile run	4-mile run	Rest	15-mile run	60-min cross
11	Rest	4-mile run	8-mile run	4-mile run	Rest	16-mile run	60-min cross
12	Rest	4-mile run	8-mile run	5-mile run	Rest	12-mile run	60-min cross
13	Rest	4-mile run	9-mile run	5-mile run	Rest	18-mile run	60-min cross
14	Rest	5-mile run	9-mile run	5-mile run	Rest	14-mile run	60-min cross
15	Rest	5-mile run	10-mile run	5-mile run	Rest	20-mile run	60-min cross
16	Rest	5-mile run	8-mile run	4-mile run	Rest	12-mile run	60-min cross
17	Rest	4-mile run	6-mile run	3-mile run	Rest	8-mile run	60-min cross
18	Rest	3-mile run	4-mile run	2-mile run	Rest	Rest	Marathon

MARATHON: NOVICE 2

Novice 2 takes you one step up from Novice 1. Do it only if you have been running more than a few months, maybe with some racing experience. The long run mileage is slightly higher, with pace runs on some Wednesdays.

Week	Mon	Tue	Wed	Thu	Fri	Sat	Sun
1	Rest	3-mile run	5-mile pace	3-mile run	Rest	8-mile run	60-min cross
2	Rest	3-mile run	5-mile run	3-mile run	Rest	9-mile run	60-min cross
3	Rest	3-mile run	5-mile pace	3-mile run	Rest	6-mile run	60-min cross
4	Rest	3-mile run	6-mile pace	3-mile run	Rest	11-mile run	60-min cross
5	Rest	3-mile run	6-mile run	3-mile run	Rest	12-mile run	60-min cross
6	Rest	3-mile run	6-mile pace	3-mile run	Rest	9-mile run	60-min cross
7	Rest	4-mile run	7-mile pace	4-mile run	Rest	14-mile run	60-min cross
8	Rest	4-mile run	7-mile run	4-mile run	Rest	15-mile run	Half marathon
9	Rest	4-mile run	7-mile pace	4-mile run	Rest	Rest	60-min cross
10	Rest	4-mile run	8-mile pace	4-mile run	Rest	17-mile run	60-min cross
11	Rest	5-mile run	8-mile run	5-mile run	Rest	18-mile run	60-min cross
12	Rest	5-mile run	8-mile pace	5-mile run	Rest	13-mile run	60-min cross
13	Rest	5-mile run	5-mile pace	5-mile run	Rest	19-mile run	60-min cross
14	Rest	5-mile run	8-mile run	5-mile run	Rest	12-mile run	60-min cross
15	Rest	5-mile run	5-mile pace	5-mile run	Rest	20-mile run	60-min cross
16	Rest	5-mile run	4-mile pace	5-mile run	Rest	12-mile run	60-min cross
17	Rest	4-mile run	3-mile run	4-mile run	Rest	8-mile run	60-min cross
18	Rest	3-mile run	2-mile run	Rest	Rest	2-mile run	Marathon

MARATHON: INTERMEDIATE 1

The major difference between intermediate and novice programs is that you do back-to-back runs on the weekend: a run at marathon pace Saturday and a long run at a slower pace on Sunday. And two 20-milers at peak training.

Week	Mon	Tue	Wed	Thu	Fri	Sat	Sun
1	60-min cross	3-mile run	5-mile run	3-mile run	Rest	5-mile pace	8-mile run
2	60-min cross	3-mile run	5-mile run	3-mile run	Rest	5-mile run	9-mile run
3	60-min cross	3-mile run	5-mile run	3-mile run	Rest	5-mile pace	6-mile run
4	60-min cross	3-mile run	6-mile run	3-mile run	Rest	6-mile pace	11-mile run
5	60-min cross	3-mile run	6-mile run	3-mile run	Rest	6-mile run	12-mile run
6	60-min cross	3-mile run	5-mile run	3-mile run	Rest	6-mile pace	9-mile run
7	60-min cross	4-mile run	7-mile run	4-mile run	Rest	7-mile pace	14-mile run
8	60-min cross	4-mile run	7-mile run	4-mile run	Rest	7-mile run	15-mile run
9	60-min cross	4-mile run	5-mile run	4-mile run	Rest	Rest	Half marathon
10	60-min cross	4-mile run	8-mile run	4-mile run	Rest	8-mile pace	17-mile run
11	60-min cross	5-mile run	8-mile run	5-mile run	Rest	8-mile run	18-mile run
12	60-min cross	5-mile run	5-mile run	5-mile run	Rest	8-mile pace	13-mile run
13	60-min cross	5-mile run	8-mile run	5-mile run	Rest	5-mile pace	20-mile run
14	60-min cross	5-mile run	5-mile run	5-mile run	Rest	8-mile run	12-mile run
15	60-min cross	5-mile run	8-mile run	5-mile run	Rest	5-mile pace	20-mile run
16	60-min cross	5-mile run	6-mile run	5-mile run	Rest	4-mile pace	12-mile run
17	60-min cross	4-mile run	5-mile run	4-mile run	Rest	3-mile run	8-mile run
18	60-min cross	3-mile run	4-mile run	Rest	Rest	2-mile run	Marathon

MARATHON: INTERMEDIATE 2

More mileage. That's the biggest difference between Intermediate 2 and
Intermediate 1. Three 20-milers. This is definitely an endurance-based
program.

Week	Mon	Tue	Wed	Thu	Fri	Sat	Sun
1	60-min cross	3-mile run	5-mile run	3-mile run	Rest	5-mile pace	10-mile run
2	60-min cross	3-mile run	5-mile run	3-mile run	Rest	5-mile run	11-mile run
3	60-min cross	3-mile run	6-mile run	3-mile run	Rest	6-mile pace	8-mile run
4	60-min cross	3-mile run	6-mile run	3-mile run	Rest	6-mile pace	13-mile run
5	60-min cross	3-mile run	7-mile run	3-mile run	Rest	7-mile run	14-mile run
6	60-min cross	3-mile run	7-mile run	3-mile run	Rest	7-mile pace	10-mile run
7	60-min cross	4-mile run	8-mile run	4-mile run	Rest	8-mile pace	16-mile run
8	60-min cross	4-mile run	8-mile run	4-mile run	Rest	8-mile run	17-mile run
9	60-min cross	4-mile run	9-mile run	4-mile run	Rest	Rest	Half marathon
10	60-min cross	4-mile run	9-mile run	4-mile run	Rest	9-mile pace	19-mile run
11	60-min cross	5-mile run	10-mile run	5-mile run	Rest	10-mile run	20-mile run
12	60-min cross	5-mile run	6-mile run	5-mile run	Rest	6-mile pace	12-mile run
13	60-min cross	5-mile run	10-mile run	5-mile run	Rest	10-mile pace	20-mile run
14	60-min cross	5-mile run	6-mile run	5-mile run	Rest	6-mile run	12-mile run
15	60-min cross	5-mile run	10-mile run	5-mile run	Rest	10-mile pace	20-mile run
16	60-min cross	5-mile run	8-mile run	5-mile run	Rest	4-mile pace	12-mile run
17	60-min cross	4-mile run	6-mile run	4-mile run	Rest	4-mile run	8-mile run
18	60-min cross	3-mile run	4-mile run	Rest	Rest	2-mile run	Marathon

MARATHON: ADVANCED 1

Advanced 1 offers a shift in focus. Welcome to speedwork, a blend on Thursdays of hill training, tempo runs, and interval running. Unless you have done speedwork in the "off season," I recommend you don't start now.

Week	Mon	Tue	Wed	Thu	Fri	Sat	Sun
1	3-mile run	5-mile run	3-mile run	3 × hill	Rest	5-mile pace	10-mile run
2	3-mile run	5-mile run	3-mile run	30-min. tempo	Rest	5-mile run	11-mile run
3	3-mile run	6-mile run	3-mile run	4 × 800	Rest	6-mile pace	8-mile run
4	3-mile run	6-mile run	3-mile run	4 x hill	Rest	6-mile pace	13-mile run
5	3-mile run	7-mile run	3-mile run	35-min. tempo	Rest	7-mile run	14-mile run
6	3-mile run	7-mile run	3-mile run	5 × 800	Rest	7-mile pace	10-mile run
7	3-mile run	8-mile run	4-mile run	5 × hill	Rest	8-mile pace	16-mile run
8	3-mile run	8-mile run	4-mile run	40-min. tempo	Rest	8-mile run	17-mile run
9	3-mile run	9-mile run	4-mile run	6 × 800	Rest	Rest	Half mara-thon
10	3-mile run	9-mile run	4-mile run	6 × hill	Rest	9-mile pace	19-mile run
11	4-mile run	10-mile run	5-mile run	45-min. tempo	Rest	10-mile run	20-mile run
12	4-mile run	6-mile run	5-mile run	7 × 800	Rest	6-mile pace	12-mile run
13	4-mile run	10-mile run	5-mile run	7 × hill	Rest	10-mile pace	20-mile run
14	5-mile run	6-mile run	5-mile run	45-min. tempo	Rest	6-mile run	12-mile run

15	5-mile run	10-mile run	5-mile run	8 × 800	Rest	10-mile pace	20-mile run
16	5-mile run	8-mile run	5-mile run	6 × hill	Rest	4-mile pace	12-mile run
17	4-mile run	6-mile run	4-mile run	30-min. tempo	Rest	4-mile run	8-mile run
18	3-mile run	4 × 400	2-mile run	Rest	Rest	2-mile run	Marathon

MARATHON: ADVANCED 2

The ultimate marathon training program. Advanced 2 offers speedwork on 2 days: Tuesday and Thursday. Still seeking improvement? You can add mileage to increase the difficulty, which may mean going to double workouts on some days.

Week	Mon	Tue	Wed	Thu	Fri	Sat	Sun
1	3-mile run	3 × hill	3-mile run	30-min. tempo	Rest	5-mile pace	10-mile run
2	3-mile run	30-min. tempo	3-mile run	3-mile pace	Rest	5-mile run	11-mile run
3	3-mile run	4 × 800	3-mile run	30-min. tempo	Rest	6-mile pace	8-mile run
4	3-mile run	4 × hill	3-mile run	35-min. tempo	Rest	6-mile pace	13-mile run
5	3-mile run	5 × 800	3-mile run	3-mile pace	Rest	7-mile run	14-mile run
6	3-mile run	5 × 800	3-mile run	35-min. tempo	Rest	7-mile pace	10-mile run
7	3-mile run	5 × hill	4-mile run	40-min. tempo	Rest	8-mile pace	16-mile run
8	3-mile run	40-min. tempo	4-mile run	3-mile pace	Rest	8-mile run	17-mile run
9	4-mile run	6 × 800	4-mile run	40-min. tempo	Rest	Rest	Half marathon
10	3-mile run	6 × hill	4-mile run	45-min. tempo	Rest	9-mile pace	19-mile run
11	4-mile run	45-min. tempo	5-mile run	4-mile pace	Rest	10-mile run	20-mile run
12	4-mile run	7 × 800	5-mile run	45-min. tempo	Rest	6-mile pace	12-mile run
13	4-mile run	7 × hill	5-mile run	50-min. tempo	Rest	10-mile pace	20-mile run
14	5-mile run	45-min. tempo	5-mile run	5-mile pace	Rest	6-mile run	12-mile run
15	5-mile run	8 × 800	5-mile run	40-min. tempo	Rest	10-mile pace	20-mile run

16	5-mile run	6 × hill	5-mile run	30-min. tempo	Rest	4-mile pace	12-mile run
17	4-mile run	30-min. tempo	4-mile run	4-mile pace	Rest	4-mile run	8-mile run
18	3-mile run	4 × 400	3-mile run	Rest	Rest	2-mile run	Marathon

ACKNOWLEDGMENTS

Cooldown: No Book Gets Written
Without a Lot of Support

Thanks to all who contributed to the success of this book.

Marathon: The Ultimate Training Guide, now in its fifth edition, has grown in breadth and depth because of hundreds, perhaps thousands, of people. If this is the textbook for the marathoning age——and I think it is—I owe thanks to all of them, coaches and runners, too many to name.

The first edition, in 1993, owed its expertise to my own successful career as a runner and sometime coach, but also to more than fifty coaches who returned questionnaires sharing their ideas and training methods. You still will find quotes from many of those coaches scattered through this edition.

In the half-dozen years between the first and second editions, I became a training consultant to the Chicago Marathon, thanks to race director Carey Pinkowski. My duties included working with the Chicago Area Running Association's Marathon Training Class, which grew from several hundred to several thousand runners under the leadership of Brian

Piper and Bill Fitzgerald and later Tom Moran. Working with the class unquestionably helped expand my knowledge.

For the third edition, I called on my Internet friends, the so-called V-Teamers—those who participated in my Virtual Training Bulletin Boards, asking me questions and helping me answer the questions of others. The fourth and now fifth editions continue my relationship with runners both online and in person. It can truly be said that we are all in this together, and I continue to be amazed at how readily runners support each other, providing advice and guidance. This book certainly celebrates the closeness of the community of runners.

Thanks also to my editors at *Runner's World* and in the Rodale book division, beginning with David Willey and John Atwood at the magazine offices in Emmaus, Pennsylvania; also my editor, Shannon Welch, and Stephanie Knapp in the Rodale offices in New York City. While Stephanie and I were working together—sending emails back and forth—making sure my writing and Shannon's editing matched the very detailed Rodale style book, Stephanie was using one of my training programs to prepare for a half marathon in Brooklyn. Others involved in the production of this book include Chris Rhoads, Amy King, and Lois Hazel.

Between the fourth and fifth editions, Rodale sold its magazine division, including *Runner's World*, to Hearst, and its book division to Penguin Random House, whose editor Michele Eniclerico inherited me as an author. Others working on this fifth edition were: designers Stephanie Huntwork and Meighan Cavanaugh, cover designer Sarah Horgan, production editor Patricia Shaw, and production manager Jessica Heim.

Angela Miller, my agent, also has endured through the first, second, third, and fourth editions of *Marathon: The Ultimate Training Guide*, both negotiating contracts and offering advice. My continuing thanks to her.

A special thanks to Nancy Clark, RD, a Boston-area dietitian, the author of *Nancy Clark's Sports Nutrition Guidebook*, also a good friend and source over the years. So much quackery exists in the field of nutrition that I did not trust myself when it came to revising and updating two key chapters. Nancy worked with me to ensure that Chapter 18, "The

Distance Runner's Diet," and Chapter 21, "Drinking on the Run," met Rodale's standards for being current and accurate.

If there is a single best source for this and many of my other books, it would be *Runner's World*'s Amby Burfoot—more than an editor, also a very close friend, along with his wife, Cristina Negron. Amby and I first met in 1965 at a small race in Warren, Rhode Island. I was at the top of my game, while Amby (who three years later would win the Boston Marathon) was not yet ready for prime time. This was in the era before prize money; New England races often offered merchandise for prizes. Traveling with my wife, Rose, and our three children, Kevin, David, and Laura, we had no room in a midsize car for any of the larger prizes. Reluctantly, I settled on a Timex watch for my first-place prize. Amby, who had finished second, claimed the combination barbecue grill and rotisserie that Rose would have loved if we could have figured out a way to transport it home to Indiana. The watch and grill are long gone, but our friendship with Amby has endured. If I need a good quote or a lead to some expert, Amby Burfoot is the first person I contact.

Rose never got that grill, but our love has endured. In addition to being husband and wife for more than a half century, we also are business partners. Without her constant assistance, we might not have sold close to a quarter million copies of *Marathon: The Ultimate Training Guide*, nor would there be this fifth edition. Rose also serves me as "last read" for all the articles and books I have submitted to various editors over the years.

Thanks to Rose and to all of you who have contributed to *Marathon: The Ultimate Training Guide*, a book that has led so many runners to the start lines and (most important) finish lines of marathons all over the world.

INDEX